CHAIR YOGA FOR SENIORS OVER 60

Fully Illustrated and Video Guide With 50+ Poses, 4 Complete Routines and a 28-Day Challenge To Elevate Your Health and Weight Loss With Quick and Easy Seated Exercises

Claire Parker

TABLE OF CONTENTS

1. Mountain Pose pag.24	2. Head and Neck Stretching pag.25	3. Shoulders Stretching pag.26	4. Wrists Stretching pag.27	5. Feet Stretching pag.28	1. Modified Cat-and-Cow (Marjaryasana-Bitilasana) pag.29
2. Twisting (Parivrtta Sukhasana) pag.30	3. Side-Bending pag.31	4. Ankle Stretching pag.32	5. Lifting Legs pag.33	6. Quadriceps and Hamstrings Stretching pag.34	7. Seated Butterfly with Yoga Block (Badha Konasana) pag.35
8. Hugging Knees pag.36	9. Interlocked Fingers and Back Bending pag.37	10. Seated Eagle Pose (Garudasana) pag.38	11. Seated Forward Bend pag.39	12. Seated Forward Bend With Two Chairs pag.40	13. Seated Child Pose (Adho Mukha Virasana) pag.41
14. Modified Downward Facing Dog (Adho Mukha Svanasana) pag.42	15. Modified Chair Pose (Utkatasana) pag.43	16. Seated Warrior I pag.44	17. Seated Warrior II Pag.45	18. Seated Reverse Warrior / Warrior III pag.46	19. Seated Humble Warrior pag.47

Yoga is not about touching your toes. It is what you learn on the way down.
—Jigar Gor

Nowadays, many have recognized that yoga is more than just a physical activity to flex the muscles of the body; it also forms a vital component of a healthy lifestyle. This, along with a surge of awareness in society regarding the importance of overall wellness, has popularized yoga practice even more. Due to its widespread appeal, more and more people are interested in giving yoga a try and eventually adopting it into their fitness regimen. While this is basically a good thing, as wider communities are benefiting from it, this trend has also spawned myths that make some individuals hesitant to take the plunge.

We can easily search for—or even be exposed to—content about yoga on the internet. With just a few clicks, we are shown tons of visuals of yogis performing beautiful yoga moves in the blink of an eye. On one hand, this could serve as motivation, especially for young people who are in good shape, to practice consistently until they can perform a variety of advanced yoga positions. Unfortunately, the tendency to glamorize aesthetics and hyper-flexibility often excludes the elderly, people with disabilities, or anyone who currently has a limited range of motion due to illness or post-surgical procedures from reaping the benefits of practicing yoga.

CHAIR YOGA: AN ATTEMPT TO MAKE YOGA MORE ACCESSIBLE TO AS MANY PEOPLE AS POSSIBLE

Yoga is much richer and deeper than just touching your toes or standing with your head down. At its core, yoga is an attempt to harmonize your mind, body, and soul. It's about being mindful to the present moment, acknowledging and being grateful of every breath we take, as well as having control over our emotion and thoughts. That is why a comprehensive yoga session must comprise breathing techniques, stretching, poses, and then relaxation or meditation. When each of these aspects is executed effectively in their respective proportions, we are actively cultivating focus and patience—something that eventually will lead us to reach the deeper state of consciousness. More than just a spiritual term, this level of depth will guide you to discover new insights about yourself and the world around you. Exploring this can help you gain clarity on the values you want to defend, the path you wish to pursue in life, the thoughts that have held you back, and the kind of relationship you aspire to have. Ultimately, you remain steadfast and unaffected by external events beyond your control, as you have discovered inner strength.

In this understanding, people will realize that there are no barriers preventing people from benefiting from yoga. Regardless of your flexibility levels, there are always ways to accommodate your circumstances. And this is where chair yoga plays its role. Even people in wheelchairs or with restricted mobility might benefit from practicing yoga while seated. This modified yoga practice is generally appropriate for anyone wishing to take a break from office work or who plans to regularly engage in mild exercise at home safely without direct supervision from a trainer or instructor.

With relatively simple movements, chair yoga is relatively easy to follow and can be done anywhere by anyone. For those who are busy and don't have much time to spare for a full yoga session, you can modify it so that you don't have to spend more than 10 minutes.

By having the flexibility to adjust the sequence based on what time you have at your disposal, this can be an excellent solution for anyone who has been trapped in a sedentary lifestyle. In this modern pace of life, most people in their productive age have to spend most of the time sitting on a chair or engaging in other passive activities, whether it's due to long hours at the office, commuting a long route, or just being glued to screens and enjoying shows from popular video on-demand platforms.

Still relevant to its inclusivity, chair yoga also breaks the deeply rooted stereotype that saying fitness is a luxury. The first thing that crosses most people's minds in relation to fitness is going to the gym to run a marathon. While both offer a lot of benefits, not everyone has the capability, either in terms of time or stamina, to do that. That is why, when you can exercise without having to leave your home, your favorite television series, or even your wheelchair, everyone is empowered to get rid of muscle stiffness and improve their overall wellness in the gentlest way possible.

A LIFE-ALTERING MOMENT THAT DROVE ME TO WRITE THIS BOOK

For me, sharing these viewpoints with you is about more than simply enlightening others about the miraculous transformations that yoga can make; it's also about an intimate encounter that ultimately inspired me to write this book. I never really cared about the dangers of sedentary living until I had to spend months in the hospital roughly five years ago, shortly after I just celebrated my 30th birthday.

Even though exercise was not an activity that came to mind, I never felt any significant pain or illness other than the occasional muscle stiffness. Thus, facing the fact that I had to spend some time trying all sorts of treatments at the hospital rather than casually hanging out with my friends or doing my hobbies was a reality check that took me aback. The pain and regret for not putting my health first pushed me to realize that I had to take action if I didn't want to be stuck in this predicament forever. That fueled me to take a degree in Sports Science and Wellness Management. I also revisited my old habits to see where could I make changes. At that moment, I knew that not only did I need to eat a healthier diet or reduce my alcohol consumption, but I also needed to regulate my stress and engage in activities that would make me calmer. Until I finally got acquainted with yoga, my savior to have a better quality of life.

WHAT THIS BOOK OFFERS YOU

I want the positive effects of my yoga routine to extend beyond myself. With my degree and career in sports and health, as well as my extensive experience of practicing yoga, I want to spread my knowledge in yoga and comprehensive wellness in general, especially to groups of people who have been marginalized in health topics for so long, simply because they are unable to move freely.

There are 40 chair yoga moves that have been meticulously curated and structured to accommodate beginners to intermediates. All poses are accompanied by some modification tips to reduce and amp up the intensities, so you can do those poses safely but also stay motivated to challenge your body to the best of your ability. These variations are not only essential to keep you stick with your workout commitment but also to diversify the muscles that are being targeted to be stretched and trained.

The mission to provide inspiration and practical resources for people looking for overall wellness is also aligned with the vision of Balanced Livings Books, the publishing company in which this book is published. They have diligently selected content to guarantee that only high-quality books reach readers as a result of their devotion to delivering reliable sources on physically active and healthy lifestyles. This cannot be taken lightly, as ensuring credible information backed by expert research is crucial to the validity of the information provided.

Through seven chapters, you will be guided to debunk the myths and deeply delve into the benefits surrounding chair yoga. Before starting any routine, you will also be directed to make intentions and do some breathing techniques. At the end of the 28-day challenge, in which you will find the more thorough information in the last chapter, you will notice that gaining independence from flexibility and confidence in your bodily foundation are something that is possible to achieve, regardless of where you start.

Another beneficial feature that makes me very proud in this manuscript is that every movement and sequence are incorporated with visual guidance through numerous videos recorded by me. In addition to the text-based explanations, these videos will be very useful to help you understand what position you should start from and how to move each step until you can perform the pose well and safely. By scanning the QR codes you find in Chapters 4 and 5, you will get lifetime access to those videos, which you can always refer back to whenever and wherever you need guidance.

SCAN ME

For starters, scan this QR code to get a glimpse of how to use all the videos provided in this book and—among all the benefits—how they will help you get through chair yoga practice.

Scan the QR code to watch the pose video or enter the following URL in your browser: https://balancedlivingbooks.com/chair-yoga-video-presentation

Now, let's jump to the first chapter to take a deeper look on the benefits, what to prepare before starting your practice, and some safety precautions.

A GIFT FOR YOU

We value you and want to provide you with all the tools you need to to improve your physical healthy. Because of this, we've put together a gift pack to help getting a happier and healthier lifestyle! To access your gift that contains:

1. Your audiobook
2. Video files to download so you can work out offline
3. Fitness tracker

Scan the QR code below. Alternatively, send us an email to info@balancedlivingbooks.com using the magic word GIFT-CHAIR YOGA FOR SENIORS.

SCAN ME

CHAPTER 1
CHAIR YOGA—THE BENEFITS AND SOME PREPARATIONS TO DO

Start where you are, use what you have, do what you can.
—Arthur Ashe

As the name implies, chair yoga is a gentle variation of yoga that enables yogis to use one (sometimes two) chair to support their balance while lowering the risk of falling and other possible injuries. As part of a subset of the broader category called "adaptive yoga," this modification was invented in 1982 by a certified Kripalu Yoga instructor, Lakshmi Voelker-Binder, to accommodate people with particular physical limitations, especially the elderly community, who are struggling with arthritis and osteoporosis that make them unable to go down to the floor easily.

Nowadays, due to its broad benefits, everyone is welcome to benefit from practicing chair yoga, regardless of their physical fitness. However, all movements mentioned in this book are specifically designed to be inclusive of seniors and those who have a limited range of motion. This includes wheelchair users and those who are still recovering after injuries or have undergone surgeries.

Aside from those who have medical concerns, chair yoga can be extremely helpful for working people who barely have time to go to the gym, even though they are actually relatively healthy. The fact that you don't need to get up from your chair makes this exercise suitable to be done during a lunch break or any short window you have. Later on in this book, there is sequence you can do in just 10 minutes. In this way, doing workouts and pursuing a healthier body is within reach of everyone, no matter how busy or stiff you are.

In this chapter, we will take a detailed look at the physical and psychological benefits of doing yoga on seated position. Also, we will prepare ourselves by learning the safety precautions and assessing our health to make sure that practice can be done safely. Now, let's open the discussion by debunking one most widespread misunderstanding about chair yoga: Does "stretching" on a chair really have benefits for people?

MORE THAN "JUST" STRETCHING

Chair yoga is indeed classified as a low-impact workout that emphasizes safe movements. Unfortunately, some people doubt its benefits, perceiving it as mere mild stretching without significant impact on the body. The simplicity of the poses often leads people to assume that this variation wouldn't be able to keep up as their bodies become accustomed to these "basic" poses. In fact, despite the fact that the posture has been altered to make it simpler than when performed on a mat, chair yoga still demands strength and good coordination, making it not just a passive activity.

Stretching, in principle, offers plenty of benefits. It lubricates joints, improves blood flow, increase flexibility, and lengthens and strengthen muscles that may rarely be stimulated. However, when you are doing a full session of chair yoga, the benefits extend beyond just stretching.

BETTER POSTURE, IMPROVED SLEEP, AND MORE FLEXIBILITY

According to research conducted by McCaffrey et al. (2019), chair yoga is proven to help older individuals dealing with osteoarthritis in their lower extremities. That experiment revealed that engaging in chair yoga for at least 16 sessions across eight weeks has been proven to improve their gait, posture, range of motion, and physical abilities to do daily activities. This enhancement also led to a better sleep cycle and alleviated pain in the muscles that were usually uncomfortable while undergoing daily activities. In terms of sleep improvement, surprisingly, another study (Wang & Boros, 2019) indicates that low to moderate at-home exercise—rather than intense, rigorous exercise—has a greater impact on quality of sleep. Those benefits have opened opportunities for a different group of people to gain something from chair yoga. Those who have functional mobility but have been struggling to mend their poor sleeping habits may give this low-impact exercise a try.

IMPROVING MENTAL HEALTH

Other benefits that have been associated with yoga are lessening stress and fostering self-love—all things related to mental health. According to a systematic review carried out by Wang and Szabo (2020), this psychological benefit isn't exclusive to traditional yoga but also includes other variations, including chair-based yoga. Adult individuals who practiced at least once a week for three consecutive months realized positive changes in stress and panic management, as well as improved mood (Tew et al., 2017).

In addition to the benefits associated with slow pace, the versatility of poses enables people to modify them in order to amp up the intensity levels if practicing the basic motion no longer feels challenging. Due to its significant impact in improving range of motion, yogis will feel better after a few months of routine practice. On one hand, they will soon come to terms with the fact that they need something more to keep up with the improvement, while also admitting that their limitations make them unable to go down to the floor yet. In this case, you are advised to do more core-strengthening poses to activate abs and arms muscles, as well as enhance stamina and endurance.

WEIGHT LOSS

If practicing core muscles through chair yoga is within reach, then how about losing weight? Yes! Some poses are good to incorporate into a weight-loss routine, especially those that target core muscles. However, there are several things to note. In general, losing weight safely and permanently requires a healthy lifestyle that includes more than just exercise. A balanced diet, regular sleep patterns, and adequate hydration are among the habits that are crucial to sustaining an ideal weight program. Managing your stress and having the moral support of those around you also help. For instance, high stress can quickly result in impulsive eating, sleep deprivation, or reluctance to break the sedentary vicious cycle.

In terms of a weight-loss exercise regimen, chair yoga can be a wise alternative due to its ability to burn calories and tone the muscles without applying pressure to lower limbs' joints. Since the majority of the movement is centered on the torso, it is easier to burn fat and tone muscles in the upper body. Furthermore, in the long term, its calm sensation can better regulate cortisol, the hormone that controls stress. When cortisol levels are high, muscular mass is lost and visceral fat (fat that resides in the abdominal area and can clog arteries) is gained.

In Chapter 5, we will provide a specific chair yoga routine for those who intend to lose weight. Most postures will be focus on strengthening core muscles, especially abdominal power, with some flexibility training to balance. This combination is essential because the more flexible you are, the more likely you are able to do more advanced and powerful poses that lead to weight-loss.

SAFETY PRECAUTION

Like any other physical activity, it is important to take safety precautions, no matter how simple the movements are. There are a few points to prepare for before starting and keep in mind throughout the session:

1.   Focus the mind only on the movement and rhythm of the breath.

Focusing on the breath and movement is the very foundation of doing yoga safely. For instance, panting breathing is one of the first signs your body sends when you extend your muscles past their capacity. When you sense that your body is trembling, this is another subtle sign that shouldn't be disregarded. Without awareness of your own body, there is a potential that you will either dismiss or be late to recognize these signs. If the latter happens, then the possibility is the tissue damage has already occurred before you finally stop exercising.

2. Sit up straight without slouching, unless the movement requires you to bend your back.

Beyond just a posture issue, an unaligned spine negatively affects your breathing. When your torso is slouched backward, you put tension on your chest and reduce your lungs' capacity to store and release air while breathing. This prevents you from taking a deep breath, increases the risk of other respiratory issues, and affects how safely you perform each pose. The more you slouch, the harder your muscles must work to balance your torso by constricting in body areas where they shouldn't. When this happens near a nerve, there is a chance that the pressure will pinch the nerve, exacerbating your existing pain or creating a new one in your supposed healthy tissue.

3. Knowing the difference between feeling pain and normal discomfort.

If you don't get used to moving your body, you will notice a slight discomfort when you stretch your muscles. Especially during poses that require balance and core strength, you may feel a little bit of trembling around your abs, arms, and thighs. In general, this is normal, as your body is signaling that the muscles are working. After all, working out requires effort, and this isn't always comfortable at first. However, there are some common symptoms that can be an indicator that the exercise you are doing may be beyond your body's capacity. For example, no workout should leave you with intense, stabbing pain, numbness, shaking violently, or other painful sensations like burning and stinging like an electrocution. When you do stretch, be careful if somehow the sensation is felt on the bones rather than the muscles or joints. Especially when you elevate the intensity more than you used to and you feel nausea and/or dizziness, that's probably signals for you to stop the exercise immediately. Go back to neutral position, get some rest, and hydrate. If your condition doesn't get better, it's best to consult with your physician.

4. When in doubt, keep in mind that doing no harm is always more important than achievements.

When you are still getting to know your body and learning how far it can go, it's not always easy to determine which pain should be tolerated or not. Whenever you feel doubtful, remember that respecting and taking care of your body is way more crucial than pursuing any achievement for being able to accomplish certain advanced poses.

5. Don't skip warm-ups.

Lengthening your muscle when it's still cold and stiff can be dangerous. When you warm up actively, you prepare your muscles by getting oxygen and blood flowing. As the blood and oxygen flow smoothly, the body temperature will rise and the heart rate will increase gradually. This helps reduce the stress on the heart during an exercise session. Psychologically, warming up can also lead the mind to focus and synchronize with the body's movements.

FREQUENTLY ASKED QUESTIONS AND ESSENTIAL HEALTH ASSESSMENTS

1. Are there any contraindications?

Consult your doctor first if you recently fell and fractured any bones, have a history of heart illness, glaucoma, high blood pressure, or severe respiratory issues.

2. What if my back is too stiff?

As long as you are cautious and mindful of your body, practicing chair yoga can be an excellent method to loosen stiffness and alleviate back pain. Strengthening and stretching are what your stiff back requires the most, and chair yoga is designed to provide just that.

Keep in mind to follow the proper steps of every posture. Almost every yoga pose requires you to lengthen your spine first before moving to the next step, either twisting or bending, to ensure that your torso has enough range of movement to do the movement. Not only does it reduce the risk of injuries, but it allows you to practice with comfort and increases the possibility for reaching a deeper stretch.

3. Can I do this if I just had surgery?

In general, gentle stretching while seated on a chair is safe for those who are conducting post-op recovery. As long as your surgeons gave you permission, this truly helps you regain your endurance, muscle mass, flexibility, and posture. Additionally, the calming and unwinding aspects of yoga itself can improve your mood and lessen the stress you experience as a result of the medical procedure. It might also benefit your practice to modify the poses using some supports, such as yoga blocks, straps, or an additional chair. This type of workout is often safe three to twelve months after surgery, though this can vary depending on the treatment and the person's health. Another consideration is to avoid straining the area where your surgery was performed and to stay away from challenging postures until you are well enough to increase the intensity.

4. Do I have to be very flexible?

In line with the spirit of chair yoga, this workout is accessible and inclusive for people regardless of their flexibility levels. In fact, it is an ideal option before trying other more rigorous variations on mat due to its low impact and safe poses.

However, keep in mind that alleviating stiff muscles and increasing flexibility are not instant processes. Depending on your starting point, it may take several weeks, months, or even years to achieve the significant transformation you desire. Instead of fixating on the end goal or the vision of what your body should achieve, approach yoga as a lifelong journey that promotes health, patience, mindfulness, and body awareness. Transformation isn't always physical; sometimes, a different perspective on how you see yourself and everything around you is also an essential milestone that is worth being grateful for.

5. Are there certain poses that I should avoid if I have osteoarthritis?

Even though chair yoga was created to accommodate those who have a history of osteoarthritis, that doesn't mean that all poses have the same level of risk. Generally speaking, it's best to leave poses that engage your spine too much, since they can be extremely dangerous for the brittle bone structure. These include any movement involving twisting (including rotating your waist and side bending) and bending forward (spinal flexion). Choose ones that allow your back to sit up straight throughout the sessions. In addition, avoid core-strength poses that require you to squeeze your abdomen as well. Get used to basic poses first before planning to increase the intensity.

THE IDEAL CHAIR TO USE
AND ADDITIONAL PROPS YOU MAY NEED

You might have noticed that some sports stores sell specialized chairs for yoga. Although having this will be absolutely helpful, it's important to know that you can use a regular chair you have available for your practice. Take these factors into consideration before starting to practice:

1. Make sure all four legs of the chair are the same length and remain stable when sitting on it. Sometimes, chairs with unbalanced legs or seats will wobble easily; avoid using to ensure safety.

2. Don't select a chair with wheels, as it can cause you to slip during the practice.

3. Choose the one that has a backrest. It's true that some yoga chairs are built without backrests on purpose. However, we will need a chair with sturdy backrest for practicing the poses mentioned in this book. Make sure the backrest is not wavy like an ergonomic work chair. Choose one that is straight (either with foam or a hard texture).

4. Adjust the height and width of the chair to suit the user. Choose one that allows you to sit with your knees bent 90 degrees, but the soles of your feet fully planted on the floor. For the width, choose one that accommodates your butt so that when you sit down, your foundation is fully on the seat, not flaring out to either side.

5. Pick one with only a thin foam on the seat. If the cushion is too soft and tender, you won't be able to center your sit bones properly. The ideal sitting position is when we can sit on our sit bones, not on layers of fat and muscles on our buttocks. This difference affects how steady your hips are; causing your bottom to be more prone to tilting when it should be squared and potentially leading to uneven weight distribution. Especially in poses that rely on your balance, inability to center your foundation on your sit bones can increase the risk of falling.

Beside a chair, there are some additional supplies that will help you do the poses that require deep stretching, balance, and core strength. Incorporating them aims to enhance the sequence's beginner-friendliness and prioritize safety. However, these items are entirely optional, and you can easily substitute some of them with regular household items, eliminating the need to buy anything extra.

1. Non-slip mat

Sometimes, when the floor is too slippery, you might be worried that the chair you're sitting on will slip, especially when you're doing movements that lift your legs. To avoid this, you can use an anti-slip mat to place under the chair to keep the chair legs from shifting while you are doing the postures. Usually, a rubberized mat will provide a better and stronger grip compared to the plastic ones (either a PVC or TPE mat).

2. Yoga blocks

Having a yoga block is helpful to reduce the intensity of stretching while maintaining balance and proper alignment. While it's possible to find various sizes that may be tailored specifically based on the purpose, most yoga block is 3 x 4.5 x 9 inches (roughly 7.5 x 11.5 x 23 cm). You can use any other household materials that are sturdy enough to substitute, such as stacks of thick books or folded blankets.

3. Straps

For poses that require you to touch your toes or to bring together on your back, you can use a strap to help you reach. If you don't have yoga strap, you can use belt or a towel.

4. Spare chair

Some of the poses mentioned in this book will need two chairs. You will be guided with additional explanations in Chapter 4, as there are some with specific instructions tailored to the movements to be performed. But as a starting point, these additional chairs ideally are similar in height and width to the main chair.

5. Comfortable yoga wear

It's true that one of the benefits of working out at home is that you don't have to think too much about your outfit and overall appearance. However, preparing comfortable clothes or workout activewear has many benefits, both in terms of comfort in movement and motivation. It makes you look and feel good about yourself, and it mentally gets you ready to give it your all in the chair. It will also serve as a reminder for you to continue your yoga practice each time you spot the clothing hanging.

PREPARING AN IDEAL SPACE FOR A PLEASANT PRACTICE

While chair yoga generally doesn't need too much space, there are some tips to prepare your room to be as comfortable and pleasant as possible. By following these, you can maximize whatever space you have—regardless of how crammed or spacious it is—to support your pleasant practice.

1. Find a quiet room if possible.

Since yoga emphasizes the importance of having a calm mind and paying attention to the present moment, it's best to practice in a place where there is no or only limited distractions. However, if avoiding noise and other distractions is not possible, don't immediately feel discouraged. Even in situations where you are unable to make changes to everything around you, you still possess the ability to govern your thoughts and feelings. When your mind starts to drift, try to pay attention only to the rhythm of your breathing and the sensations that arise when moving your body slowly.

2. Pay attention to the lighting.

Compared to exercising under artificial lights, there are a lot of added benefits to using natural lights. It helps your body get vitamin D, feel more energized, uplift your mood, and improve sleeping habits. To absorb all these benefits, exercise in the morning in a room where natural light can enter. If you find that doing exercise before bed improves your quality of sleep, try chair yoga twice a day, every day and night. In times when you are unable to spend too much time, you can concentrate more on the body parts that feel more strained and make the routine brief. Later in Chapter 5, you will get a recommendation for 10-minute yoga; use this as your go-to routine whenever you need a quick stretch.

If it's not possible to rely on natural light, you can put some lighting in the room that enhance your focus while still maintaining your calmness. Choose one that won't interfere with your meditation state by having soft hues and brightness. Alternatively, you may want to use one with adjustable light fixtures. In times when you want to practice more dynamic routines that demand strength and power, opt for bright light. Conversely, choose the warm and dim light for restorative sequences.

3. Stimulate your olfactory senses with essential oils or incense.

Aromatherapy has long been thought to help us focus better, retain mindfulness, and integrate our physical, mental, and spiritual selves. Diluting them in a burner or diffuser so you have a nice aroma in your room can help you focus, especially if you frequently struggle to do so because your mind is constantly racing. These following scents are suggested: cedarwood, patchouli, lavender, frankincense, vetiver, jasmine, chamomile, and cinnamon.

4. Use some background music.

If you find it difficult to focus on silence, selecting a suitable background music might make you feel more at ease as you concentrate. While there is no hard-and-fast rule on finding the best music for yoga, it doesn't mean that any genre or type of music will affect the ambience of your practice in the same way.

You can tailor the music based on the pace of routines you currently do. For example, the same upbeat music can uplift your mood when you are doing weight-loss or power chair yoga, yet it is too agitating for bedtime stretching that is supposed to be more calming. Once you find the music that suits your intention, organize your playlist in such a way that the dynamics build from gentle and relaxing to help you enter the meditative stage of the breathing technique, then slowly become more intense as you proceed to other more intense warm-ups and poses. Finally, wrap up with another gentle instrument as your body enters restorative poses like child pose or savasana.

5. Keep the room tidy and clean.

Maintaining the cleanliness of the space you will use to practicing yoga is the bare minimum. If you use a mat under your chair, make sure you wipe it off to remove the dirt and grease that may reduce its grip.

After learning a lot about the benefits and essential preparations before starting our yoga journey, take a look at the next chapter, as we want to discuss how to build a healthy habit that lasts. Learning how to maintain this new habit as a part of your daily life is equally vital because yoga is an ongoing process that has to be practiced consistently in order to reap advantages that last over time.

CHAPTER 2
HABITS AND MOTIVATION

And actually, it's not repetition that creates habits. It's emotions that creates habits.
—Rangan Chatterjee

Almost everyone is aware of the importance of a healthy lifestyle and how it can affect all aspects of our lives, both physically and mentally. Unfortunately, not everyone can or knows how to maintain this change so that it lasts permanently. Take a look at how many people see the new year or birthday as the perfect time of the year to set annual resolutions. Then a year later, how many of them are able to check—at least half or three-quarters—of the list, let alone all of them?

Unless you've been very disciplined with yourself, chances are we've all experienced first-hand how hard it is to let go of bad habits, despite the fact that we also realize there's no benefit to sticking with it. However, don't lose hope. By following the right steps and adopting the right mindset, we can make a healthy lifestyle a part of our daily habits—and that's our goal for this chapter.

In this chapter, we will explore practical tips to maintain a consistent workout routine. When you feel demotivated or lose sight of your goals, you can revisit this chapter for a motivational boost and regain your momentum. Additionally, we will discuss the significance of self-care and self-awareness, and how they contribute to sustaining healthy habits.

FORMING A LASTING HEALTHY HABIT

Almost everything we do in life is part of a habit, from the mundane tasks like brushing your teeth, doing laundry, making up your bed, and organizing bottles in your kitchen to something that is more technical and requires skills, such as how you do your job in a professional context or exercising hobbies like cooking, crocheting, and gardening. Most of them don't require you to analyze the situation; you just do it because that's what you always do for as long as you remember. So, what drives us to do certain things, and how to "hack" our brains to automatically become habituated to a healthy habit?

Habits are actually patterns that we develop in response to specific circumstances. They happen under three variables: a cue, an action or activity, and an incentive. A cue is the appearance of a certain condition that gives us a signal to do something. This can be in the form of a place, person, smell, scenery, time, and many more. When we notice the cue, then we will automatically do something that is associated with it. For example, when you see the sky darken, you will instinctively switch on the lamp. Then the incentive is the reward we get after fulfilling the activity. In the case of turning on the lamp, we will get a sense of security as a reward. It doesn't always come in the form of a tangible object like money or a present; instead, most of it takes abstract forms of a sense of contentment, security, answering curiosity, or even just a whim—basically every positive feeling that you feel afterward.

By understanding this concept, we have the ability to transform any negative habits into positive ones by manipulating the cue, action, and incentive. In the case of setting up a workout routine, we can strategically place our workout clothes in a visible location as a cue. Alternatively, we can set up reminders on our phones to prompt us at specific times and days to encourage consistent practice. As for the reward, picture yourself having the ability to be more independent and more comfortable with a healthier, less stiff body.

Regardless of how achievable and realistic the goal you have set, it's easy to get demotivated when you can't see the "reward" you intend in a short time. Even though you are perfectly aware that practicing a healthy habit won't offer you immediate gratification, it's tough to continue the journey when the destination is no longer in sight.

To overcome this situation and other possible scenarios that prevent you from keeping tabs on your goals, there are some practical steps you can take.

1. Set a specific yet realistic plan.

To enhance your motivation and commitment to your workout routine, it's beneficial to go beyond a generic plan of "do a workout exercise." Instead, consider specifying the day, time, and duration of each session. For instance, you could schedule leg-strengthening and twisting stretches every Tuesday, Thursday, and Saturday from 6.30 to 6.50 AM. Strive for a realistic plan that challenges you without overwhelming you from the start.

2. Keeping track of your progress in your journal or calendar.

Keeping a log of your planned activities can be incredibly satisfying, especially when dealing with habits that don't show immediate progress after a single session. Later in Chapter 6, there will be a QR code you can scan to download a track list. You can use this to solidify your healthy habit of practicing chair yoga, as well as part of your gratitude and appreciation to review how far you've come. In this manner, you will become more aware of your daily progress and be driven to stay on course.

3. Sharing your commitment with people you trust.

Sometimes, people will feel much more motivated to do something when driven by the desire to maintain an image in front of others. After setting up the realistic plan, you can ask your closest one to hold you accountable. Tell them that you are going to spend 30 minutes, three times a week, doing targeted stretching. Give them weekly updates on your accomplishments (whether you really spend that amount of time working out and how many times you miss). In times when you lose motivation to keep up the work, there is a higher chance you won't lose progress because you don't want to show others that you "failed" to meet the targets you set for yourself.

4. Set a buffer time to compensate when you are missing your plan.

Sometimes, a single moment of setback can shatter the carefully cultivated habit you've worked so hard to maintain. People often miss their targets due to unexpected events or overestimating their capabilities. Initially, you may have been confident enough to commit to exercising three times a week. However, as time went on, you realized that fatigue made it difficult to keep up, causing you to miss a session. To prevent losing motivation entirely, consider setting aside extra time or having a backup plan to anticipate such slumps. This way, you'll still have something to linger on when the main plan doesn't go as expected.

5. Enjoy the process.

Keep in mind that having a healthy habit is a lifetime journey. Regardless of how tedious it is, try your best to find something joyful during the process. You can cultivate this mindset by appreciating every milestone you have accomplished; including the gratitude to be able to lift your legs, enjoy the moment your body is drenched in nice sweat, and notice that your range of movement around your hips has improved slowly but steadily.

6. Arrange an instant reward for your progress and negative consequences.

Aside from its associated long-term benefits, you can add other rewards and impose some "consequences" that may not have a direct relationship with your new habit but are able to keep you motivated. For example, if you often feel too lazy to start exercising because you don't want to miss the new episode of your favorite TV shows, you can use this as a reward and punishment system. If you usually watch three episodes each day, cut it to only one for every planned workout session you miss. On the other hand, add one episode as a reward every time you finish your session. To make sure you comply with your own rules, tell your trusted one so they will help you be more accountable to yourself.

In addition to lack of motivation, sometimes the thing that hinders you from achieving a healthy habit is the worst-case scenario that you picture over and over time in your head. This can manifest in the fear of failure, a lack of confidence in embracing change, or a feeling of overwhelm with the continuity of the process. If this isn't addressed properly, then there is a chance that your internal fears change your perception of what is good and bad for yourself. However, there are some tips to follow to break this cycle and prevent you from drowning in your own negativity.

1. Jotting down of what occupies your mind.

Every time you feel your mind is racing, take a piece of paper and a pen. List everything that makes you afraid or that you think will hinder your way of incorporating healthy habits. After that, take a break for a few minutes and go back and read what you have listed. Break down your previous writings with the feelings behind those negative thoughts in as detail as possible. This includes any past event that may trigger your anxiety or negative news you read on social media. When you are done, try to challenge your own perspectives by listing your strengths, what tangible actions you can take to overcome those issues, and why proper preparation and complying to safety precautions isn't enough. You will realize that most fears and insecurities are more menacing in your mind than they truly are in reality.

2. Read success stories of someone who have similar circumstances.

Immerse yourself in positive stories shared by individuals who have faced similar situations. This will create a sense that you are not alone and motivate you to overcome your own barriers.

3. Admit that there is always a risk of doing something as well as doing nothing.

If you've been experiencing stiffness and difficulty moving your body for too long, maybe your biggest fear is injuries and exacerbate discomfort. Rather than denying this feeling, it's wise to admit that the risk of this thing happening has never been zero. Either way, the mindset to always be cautious and vigilant can save you from bad things because you are fully aware with yourself and your surroundings. Unfortunately, we also need to admit that doing nothing poses another set of risk that equally unpleasant. As we know, stretching through chair yoga can be one of the most ideal way to loosen your muscle and regain your flexibility. Therefore, completely avoiding these activities takes away your chance to heal and get better. In the end, your body will just feel more stiff and more sensitive to pain.

MITIGATING SOME OF THE MOST COMMON EXCUSES

Now that you know all the tricks for overcoming inner doubts and maintaining motivation, does this imply that you will be released from any excuses that might keep you from continuing your yoga practice? Evidently, not always.

Frequently, particularly in the initial days of practicing, you've come to understand the benefits of yoga but your body is still adjusting. As a result, the practice session hasn't gone as smoothly as you had hoped, either you may still need additional props to perform the simplest poses or the soreness after stretching sessions that you haven't done in long time. The point is, you have a ton of reasons to quit practicing and revert to your old behaviors. To avoid that, let's look at some of the most popular excuses and how to overcome them.

Since yoga doesn't generate progress in the short term, you need to keep doing it as a regular habit before you can see the difference. Unfortunately, people frequently hesitate to stick to the plan because they believe they don't have enough time. Actually, rather than depending on their own free time, the majority of people exercise because they set aside a specified time for it. If you think that your body can't keep up because you feel too tired, you can try to implement a five-minute examination. Try to do some warm-ups or poses until the five minutes are up on your timer. Next, evaluate yourself; are you still feeling energetic enough to go on? If so, carry on for an additional five minutes. However, stop if you start to pant excessively. It would be easier for you to ultimately increase the duration from five minutes to 10, 15, 20, or more by using this approach.

Ultimately, try to make reference to your original objective. By dedicating yourself to your personal "why," you will develop an internal drive to put all of your uncomfortable feelings aside and create a long-term focus to follow through on your plan.

HOW PRACTICING SELF-CARE MAKES YOUR HABITS LAST LONGER

Contrary to popular belief which defines "self-care" as merely activities that lift your mood, the essence of this practice actually extends beyond that. It involves nurturing yourself to achieve a harmonious balance between your responsibilities, mental well-being, and physical health. It's about synergistically ensuring that actions in one area do not compromise the others. Taking an example, dedicating time each morning to meditation can greatly enhance calmness and foster a sense of gratitude. However, without maintaining a proper balance of sufficient sleep and physical exercise, the benefits of meditation may be hindered due to drowsiness and lethargy throughout the day.

Finding this balance is crucial for maintaining healthy habits. If your daily activities leave you exhausted and stressed, you may not have the energy to do anything else that matters to your emotional and physical health. Without proper balance, even though it oftentimes becomes too delicate, you may find yourself unable to cope with life stressors and easily overwhelmed with everything around you, which can jeopardize your relationships with yourself and others.

PRACTICAL EXERCISES TO RAISE SELF-CARE AND SELF-AWARENESS

In the attempt to achieve balance, there are five aspects to cover, each consisting of example activities to do.

PHYSICAL

1. Avoid ultra-processed food and food that is high in salt, sugar, and fat.
2. Attempt to sleep at least eight hours per day.
3. Engage in a workout routine.

SPIRITUAL

1. Write a journal about three things for which you are grateful today.
2. Try a five-minute morning meditation.
3. Have a hobby that allows you to reconnect with yourself and focus on the present.

SOCIAL

1. Socialize with others and nurture your relationships with them.
2. Join a club that suits your interests.
3. Engage in conversations with friends and family, particularly those with whom you were once close but now have limited communication.

COGNITIVE

1. Read at least two pages a day from a book that you find interesting.
2. Learn and explore something new. It can be nurturing a new houseplant, learning how to solve a rubric, or doing color therapy from a coloring book for adults.

1. Learn how to manage your anger or deal with anger and frustration.

2. Talk to a therapist to deal with uncomfortable emotions that you have been unable to express for too long.

By knowing the essential "life hacks" to form a lasting habit, you can use this for the good of your body. Keep in mind to balance your efforts to establish a healthy lifestyle with some self-care and self-awareness exercises, since this is one of the keys to helping your body get accustomed to the new workouts you want to achieve. Even so, despite all the preparations you've made, there are times when you feel hesitant or worried about things you can't control. When this happens, don't feel discouraged. After all, your feelings are valid and shouldn't be brushed off. Do some tricks to unravel your busy mind, and you will notice that sometimes your mind pictures something scarier than reality. In the next chapter, we will discuss the structure of yoga practice and why all its components are what make yoga helpful to harmonize your mind, body, and soul.

CHAPTER 3
STRUCTURE OF THE PRACTICE

Move your joints every day. You have to find your own tricks. Bury your mind deep in your heart, and watch the body move by itself. —Dharma Mittra

After familiarizing yourself with the preparations, safety precautions, and tips to stay motivated for a healthy life, let's delve into the structure and components of a complete chair yoga session. In this chapter, we will explore the benefits of each component and their contribution to helping you regain a harmonious mind, body, and soul through a well-structured yoga session. Please note that specific instructions and examples will not be provided here. Instead, practical explanations and step-by-step guidance will be covered in the next chapter.

INTENTIONS

In the preceding chapter, we explored the significance of having an accountability partner to support your pursuit of a healthy habit. We can apply a similar approach in a more targeted manner by establishing intentions prior to engaging in a yoga routine. Emerging evidence suggests that this practice can influence your behavior, fostering determination and self-love as you strive to achieve your fitness goals.

According to research (Zhu et al., 2022), setting up specific intentions can instinctively positively change the behavior to be more in line with the goal to be achieved. Quite similar to the concept of habit formation, having an intention is like simulating your brain to see the workout as a cue that motivates you to really execute the plan rather than lingering on excuses or internal fears. Especially for those who initially have low motivation to break the cycle of sedentary living, having a clear intention can help them to do more exercise compared to those who don't make one.

BREATHING TECHNIQUES

Breathing is more than just an unconscious activity, and the ancient yoga tradition has acknowledged the connection between breathing and self-awareness since thousands of years ago. In Sanskrit, the term pranayama refers to breathing techniques that we use in yoga, although people can practice them anytime, anywhere they need to calm mind chatter. When engaging in yoga, this technique facilitates the transition of your mind and body into a deeper state of consciousness before proceeding with the rest of the sequence. This is an important part as we try to gradually sharpen our mindfulness by leaving behind other businesses, agendas, or thoughts that occupy our mind before entering a yoga session.

In order to enter a deeper consciousness, we are guided to breathe the "right" way. Sometimes, during moments of anxiety or panic, our breathing becomes shallower and faster. This not only increases fatigue, but also disrupts the flow of oxygen in our respiratory system. When we don't fully take in oxygen and expel carbon dioxide, our heart beats faster than normal, intensifying feelings of fatigue and anxiety, as well as decreasing pain tolerance. On the contrary, when we inhale and exhale deeply, it revitalizes and brings a sense of calmness to our body due to an increase of dopamine and endorphins, two hormones that are responsible for the feeling of happiness and a sense of well-being. Furthermore, a more balanced ratio of oxygen and carbon dioxide can help stabilize blood pressure, relax the muscles, and improve blood flow. When consistently practiced over the long term, your lung capacity will expand, and your ability to manage anger will improve.

While most pranayama promote deep, slow breathing, there are two techniques that require rapid, forceful breathing called bhastrika and kapalbhati. These exercises are highly effective for engaging the abdominal muscles, boosting overall energy levels, and promoting detoxification through respiration. You may experience an immediate increase in body temperature, which is beneficial for preparing your body to perform the poses, particularly if you aim to enhance core strength and balance control.

Slow breathing in the pranayama concept offers numerous variations to choose from with a wide range of benefits. For example, you can choose a three-part breathing if you want to train your body to be able to breathe deeper toward your abdominal cavity; people often refer to this as diaphragm breathing or belly breathing. If you're already used to shallow breathing, doing diaphragmatic breathing will make you realize how much oxygen capacity you can breathe and how it's never put to good use when we breathe short. Activating the diaphragm not only promotes calmness and manages stress, but also has a positive effect on the digestive system. Especially when practicing on an empty stomach, this technique stimulates the vagus nerve. The vagus nerve is the longest nerve in the human body, extending from the neck to the torso. It regulates various unconscious functions, such as heartbeat, blood pressure, and digestion. This stimulation improves blood flow and increases oxygen levels in the digestive organs, leading to better nutrient absorption. Additionally, activating the diaphragm has a massage-like effect on the internal organs, reducing the severity of bloating, constipation, and other bowel issues.

There are other variations that help you become more conscious of your breathing in a way that, most likely, you may only occasionally or never do. One is anuloma viloma, which allows you to breathe via one nostril at a time, and the other is kumbhaka, which involves a pause between inhaling and exhaling.

Holding your breath for a few seconds can, when done correctly, lessen your risk of inflammation, expand the lungs' cavity to inhale deeper, and preserve the functionality of your cardiovascular system. In the same vein, alternating your breath through each nostril has an invigorating effect, as your parasympathetic nervous system (PNS) becomes more relaxed. This has an advantageous influence on one's mental clarity, level of energy, and ability to concentrate. In relation to the concentration, a study (Telles et al., 2017) has showed that this pranayama helps people to be more focused without losing the sense of vigilant. Therefore, this technique is ideal for anyone who needs to better regulate their anxiousness without drifting off or losing their focus.

HANDS' POSITION WHEN PRACTICING BREATHING TECHNIQUES

While some techniques require you to place your hands in a certain way, others let you rest your hands comfortably in your lap. But there are other options available to you as well. You can do traditional yogic hands' gestures called mudras.

In Sanskrit, the word mudra means a seal or a gesture. For hundreds, or even thousands of years, people have used this hand position as a means to connect with their higher selves and divinity. This has to do with the traditional hand philosophy, which maintains that the hand is a representation of the soul, self-reflection, prayer, and meditation. Until now, this practice has still been practiced due to the belief that the tip of our fingers is connected with the fundamental elements—earth, water, fire, air, and space (often referred to ether)—that are responsible for the balance of human beings' lives. Therefore, mudras have various gestures that can be adjusted to which areas in life require more energy.

When you want to incorporate these symbolic gestures during breathing practice, there are several recommendations that are believed can enhance the spiritual and psychological effects of pranayama:

1. Chin Mudra

Try doing the chin mudra to enhance mindfulness, focus, and mental sharpness. Place your palms comfortably on your lap and bring the tips of your thumb and index finger together. Your palms should be facing upward in this position, with your thumb and forefinger in a circle and the remaining fingers relaxed and extended.

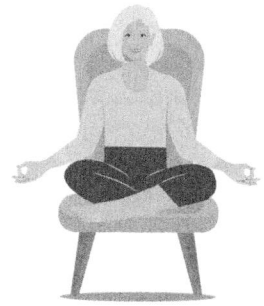

2. Anjali Mudra

This is probably the most well-known mudra. Most people associate it with praying hands, or in the context of yoga, many refer to it as the namaste pose. The conventional type of yoga, which is practiced on a mat, often incorporates this gesture into some asana like tree pose and standing mountain pose. When you gently press your palms to each other in front of your chest, we are humbled to reflect our lives at the depths of our hearts and to reconnect with the divine. Therefore, it's ideal to prepare our mind and consciousness to enter a contemplative state.

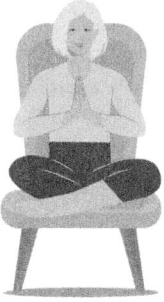

3. Bharairava and Bhairavi Mudra

If your fingers are stiff to the extent that folding them may make you uncomfortable, you can try these gestures. To do bharairava mudra, stack your right palm on top of your left one, whereas in bharairavi is the opposite, the left palm on top of your right palm. Since you can place your hands slightly below your navel or rest them on your lap in a relaxed manner, this would be a suitable choice if your arms or wrists encounter challenges in maintaining stability while in a floating Anjali mudra position. It's best to pair this gesture with deep, slow breathing techniques.

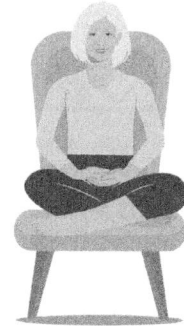

4. Ushas Mudra

Another alternative for calming mudra, in which both hands are engaged to form one gesture, is usha mudra. This gesture can help calm and stabilize you if you tend to become agitated easily over trivial things but are sluggish during the day. You can do this by loosely interlacing your fingers with both thumbs stacked on top of each other. When you press your thumbs gently, regardless of its soothing nature, the application is quite varied, and it isn't limited to a slow breathing rhythm. If you feel comfortable, you can do this while doing rapid and forceful breathing. Drag your hands until the palms gently touch your lower belly. By feeling your belly expand and deflate rapidly, you can easily focus on your breath and maintain the tempo.

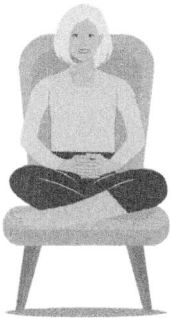

WARMING UPS

Some people mistakenly believe that since yoga is a low-impact exercise, there is no need for a warm-up because the poses themselves already mimic warm-ups. Unfortunately, this is a dangerous approach that can increase the risk of injury.

Like what we already discussed in the previous chapter, warming up in yoga is highly essential to lengthening the muscles and preparing your body to do poses that require deeper stretching and activation in targeted areas. You can also utilize this stage to evaluate the extent of your range of motion and identify the poses in the next stage that you can perform effortlessly or require modification. In the same vein, warming up makes you more aware of your body to know which parts feel stiffer and need more attention than others.

Instead of focusing on only loosening the muscles, you need to target all the joints during warm-ups. This includes stretching your neck, shoulders, wrists, fingers, ankles, toes, and hips. Do it by making a circle motion until you feel the activation. Keep in mind to always maintain your deep breathing rhythm.

POSES/POSTURES

This is perhaps the part that is most associated with the image of yoga. The physical practice in which we perform various poses and postures is called asanas in Sanskrit with the direct translation in English meaning "seat." Before the practice of yoga became widely popular, like nowadays, the term asana in ancient practice referred to the sitting position when people meditated.

For most people who initially try yoga to improve the flexibility of their muscles, it's most likely that they see asana as the key of yoga practice itself. In fact, it's just one of the eight limbs (ashtanga) of yoga that are described in the ancient scripture Patanjali's Yoga Sutras: pranayama, asana, yamas (social norms), niyamas (self-awareness), pratyahara (disconnection from the outside world), dharana (focus), dhyana (meditate) and samadhi (profound connection to spirituality).

To be able to reach the highest consciousness—samadhi—we must have a healthy physique. As a result, asana comprises of a wide range of positions and postures that explore practically all body parts, from the crown of the head to the tips of the toes. Another important aspect of asana that all yogis should remember, regardless of whatever yoga variations they practice, is the seamless integration of body movements and breathing practice. Whenever you move your body, try to keep a continuous rhythm of deep breathing.

RELAXATION AND MEDITATION

As a way to relax and collect our breath after doing asanas, we can do restorative poses like child pose and corpse pose. When practiced correctly—that is, when we don't get carried away by the flow of noisy thoughts or fall asleep—these rejuvenating positions will help you reduce muscle fatigue, stabilize blood pressure, alleviate sleep deprivation, and lessen the likelihood of headaches. Especially with the child pose, it gives you a nice stretch around lower back and hips; perfect for relieving any tension that often happens not only because of sedentary living, but also when we feel anxious or stressed.

Due to its similar benefits, child pose can be a great alternative for relaxation without having to recline your back like corpse pose. When you lean your torso forward in a relaxed manner, it helps your parasympathetic nerves to calm down as your body alters its fight-or-flight response during stress and discomfort. As a result, you will be able to wind down and watch your breath more mindfully.

In addition to promoting physical tranquility, this pose helps your body into a meditative state by allowing your senses to rest and shifting your attention to higher consciousness. With our face down and chin close to our chest, we will instinctively disregard any distractions and discomforts around us that are far beyond our control. At the same time, we will focus on our presence, stabilize the rhythm of our breath, and find it easier to control our thoughts while meditating.

Unfortunately, instead of enjoying its motionless and serene state, some people often choose to skip this stage entirely. It's best not to skip relaxation and meditation since this is the key component of yoga practice as we work to balance and settle our bodies and minds.

GRATITUDE AND APPRECIATION

Yoga's method of fostering gratefulness in each practice is what makes it an ideal exercise to develop your sense of gratitude while also strengthening your muscles. You can cultivate your gratitude in yoga through setting a specific intention that you contemplate during relaxation, meditation. or pranayama. Use this moment to reflect and show kindness for whatever your body is capable or incapable of doing during the poses.

In general, developing an attitude of appreciation is similar to forming any other healthy habit in that it involves consistent practice over time. Even though it's not always simple, especially in today's culture when perfection is the norm, once we can consistently do it, we will see a positive change in our lives. It will impact not just your mental state and self-perception, but also the quality of your established relationships with other people. This happens because, when you are happy, your body releases two chemical compounds called oxytocin and dopamine. The burst of these hormones helps strengthen your emotional bonds with others, nurture trust and openness, and foster positive feelings on other's companies. Therefore, if you find yourself having trouble developing and upholding relationships with those you value most, you might need to look at yourself and assess your gratitude levels first before thinking about the possibility that something went wrong in others.

In the context of yoga practice, appreciation and gratitude also contribute to your progress. People who are more appreciative for their lives tend to have higher resilience and self-control. This enables you to treat your body with more patience when your workout becomes taxing. It also helps you to maintain healthy habits because you will be able to more focus on what you have accomplished and the positive associations in doing the healthy things, rather than becoming bogged down in what you are lacking or how draining it feels to follow the routines.

Now, in this last part of this chapter, you have learned what the correct structure looks like according to the values that are upheld by yoga practice. The ultimate aim of yoga practice is the harmonious integration of body, mind, and spirit; this pattern exists for a reason, and adhering to it will help you get there. Each stage has a distinct role in getting your body and mind ready. Therefore, it is helpful to follow the sequence in order to transition from whatever activities you have done before yoga into a calmer state of mind and more prepared body to go through all these steps: setting an intention, practicing breathing techniques, moving your body in a series of warm-ups and asanas, winding down in relaxation and meditation, and incorporating gratitude and appreciation.

In the next chapter, we will get thorough ideas on the technicalities of practicing all aspect in this yoga structure. This includes step-by-step explanations and images of every warm-up and pose to guide you through a safe and pleasant practice. As additional resource, you will receive audio visual guidance by scanning the QR codes provided in each point.

CHAPTER 4
CHAIR YOGA—THE STEP-BY-STEP

The true purpose of yoga is to discover that aspect of your being that can never be lost.
—Deepak Chopra

Now that we have learned about the complete systematization of yoga sessions, it's time to begin the most essential part of our chair yoga journey: practice!

In this chapter, you will be guided by thorough step-by-step instructions of six breathing practices, five warm-ups, and forty poses. Furthermore, realizing that every posture and warm-up has room for adjustment and variety, this book provides you with tips to make it accessible to beginners while yet providing a sufficient level of challenge for those with increased endurance and flexibility. You will also receive guidance on how to meditate while sitting down, as well as recommendations of a weekly list of yoga intentions.

One of the book's other incredibly helpful features is that every pose is demonstrated in a video recorded by me. You have unrestricted access to this supplementary resource. Accessing this is completely optional, but I strongly advise you to do so because it provides a detailed visual guide with voice instructions, increasing your safety by ensuring that your moves are proper. You can use the camera on your smartphone to scan the QR code to view the video, or you can use your browser to input the URL that appears next to the code.

SETTING UP INTENTIONS

While the term is quite universal, yogic philosophy recognizes the concept of intentions called sankalpa as a determination that reflects what you really want and need deep down. This isn't a selfish wish that just serves a few interests that could unintentionally harm you or other people. It's also deeper than simply wishing for your future aspirations or ambitions to come true. Most of the time, our goals only concentrate on our desired state—the place where we want to be—rather than the circumstances in which we truly have a meaningful connection with ourselves.

At first, people may have tendency to find some connections between the right sankalpathings do with physical needs. Especially for individuals with physical impairments, long-term bodily discomfort, or any other restricted movements, the image of a healthy, fully functional physique may be followed by an expectation of an improved quality of life. While there is no wrong in hoping for a healthier body from routinely doing exercise, we may find something deeper that we intend to accomplish once we can delve into our inner self.

Meditation and writing in a gratitude journal can be the first, most feasible step to get the idea of your true sankalpa. Allowing your mind to attain stillness may give you different perspective on what blocks you from living a fuller, more content life. You can incorporate all these thoughts in your daily intentions every time you plan to practice yoga. Furthermore, you can also combine with something that is more practical and physical to help you tailor targeted movements that are suitable with your conditions. Let's take a look on this weekly idea:

Days	Intentions	Recommendations for targeted movements or prompts during meditation.
Monday	I want to be more patience and more compassionate with myself.	Spare more time for breathing practice. You can combine more than one pranayama at one session.
Tuesday	I desire my foundation to be steadier and more balanced.	Focus on poses that put emphasis on foundation, for example: boat pose, intense forward bend, pigeon pose, high lunge. For meditation or journaling prompts, you can start by, "What makes you restless most often?" and "What simple things happen in everyday life that make you feel more grounded?"
Wednesday	I desire to be more self-assured, embrace gratefulness, and less critical of myself.	Exercise more with poses that allow you to open your chest. Prompt examples for meditation and journaling include, "What simple activities can you do to relieve anxiety when it strikes?" and "What 10 things do I love the most from myself?"
Thursday	To welcome change, I want to preserve what I already have.	Incorporate more poses that focus on backbend and core muscle, for example: cat-and-cow pose, deep forward bend, all warrior poses, chair pose, and airplane pose. Focus your meditation and journaling sessions on questions like, "After I look back at my life for a while, what are the things that make me happy and grateful?" and "What makes you worry about the changes you currently face in life?"
Friday	I would like to worry less about the future.	Add some soothing poses to help you unwind, including downward-facing dog, goddess pose, forward bend and bridge pose.
Saturday	I desire to have stronger footing and more level shoulders.	Put more emphasis on exercises that focus on your footing and foundation, such as butterfly pose, tortoise pose, half lord of the fish pose II, and revolved goddess pose.
Sunday	I wish to mend the rift between my inner and outer selves.	Use some prompts that revolved around self-love and self-acceptance, including "What valuable trait about yourself have you recently learned?" and "What are the three endeavors you always do that are consistent with the values you most strongly hold?"

1. THE THREE-PART BREATHING (DIRGHA SWASAM)

Scan the QR code or visit this URL to watch the video pose: https://balancedlivingbooks.com/chair-yoga-video-01/

SCAN ME

INSTRUCTIONS

1. Put your right palm on your left chest and your left hand on your lower abdomen.
2. Take a deep breath from both nostrils. Your right hand should feel your chest expand, while your left hand should notice your belly gets bigger as if we were filling up a balloon.
3. Exhale slowly; feel like the air is moving upwards from the stomach, chest, and esophagus, up to both nostrils.
4. Do this technique for at least two minutes.

2. WHISPERING BREATH (UJJAYI PRANAYAMA)

Scan the QR code or visit this URL to watch the video pose: https://balancedlivingbooks.com/chair-yoga-video-02/

SCAN ME

INSTRUCTIONS

1. Start off by taking several deep breaths to get the breathing technique going.
2. Inhale deeply through your nostrils, then exhale slowly while constricting your throat. The vibration will produce a sound like snoring.

COMMON MISTAKES TO AVOID

1. Exhaling through the mouth; always inhale and exhale through your nostrils.
2. Focusing on the sound of the breath. Although it's true that the whispering noise makes this technique distinct from the others, one thing we should pay more attention to is the vibration of the throat. For this reason, just focus on the constriction of the throat. As long as it vibrates enough, it doesn't matter how loud (or silent) your breath is.

GENERAL TIPS

1. Make sure the air only passes through your nostrils by using this method without opening your lips.
2. There is no pausing between inhaling and exhaling. Since inhaling and exhaling have the same duration, there is no need to keep track of the rhythm.

3. ALTERNATE NASAL BREATHING (ANULOMA VILOMA)

Scan the QR code or visit this URL to watch the video pose: https://balancedlivingbooks.com/chair-yoga-video-03/

INSTRUCTIONS

1. Relax your body with your eyes closed and your face facing forward.
2. Place the index and middle fingers in the center of your forehead. Let the thumb close to the right nostril and the ring finger next to the left nostril.
3. In the meantime, let your left hand rest on your lap. with the palm face upward, downward, or in chin mudra position (see Chapter 3); choose the one that makes you most comfortable.
4. Press the left nostril with your ring finger.
5. Take a deep, slow breath through the right nostril.
6. Release your ring finger while pressing your right nostril with your thumb. Exhale deeply and slowly through your left nostril.
7. Deeply inhale again with your left nostril without changing fingers' position.
8. Release your thumb and exhale through right nostril.
9. Repeat the breathing technique alternately for at least two minutes. Once it is done, lower your right hand to your lap and continue the deep, steady breath.

COMMON MISTAKES TO AVOID

1. Breathing too fast and panting.
2. Forcing the air too hard, especially during exhalation.
3. Using your mouth to inhale and/or exhale; let the air flow solely through one nasal.
4. Rushingly exhaled before the chest and abdomen were filled with air during inhalation.

GENERAL TIPS

1. Attempt to exhale longer than the inhalation. You can start by counting from one to four while taking one deep breath, then release it in six counts. If this feels too easy, try to do 6-8 (six counts of inhaling and eight counts of exhaling), 8-10, or more. You are also allowed to do other, more advanced variations that let you exhale two times longer than the inhalation. This way, the tempo should be 4-8, 5-10, 6-12, and so on.
2. This technique is supposed to help slow your heartbeat. If you feel the uncontrollable tendency to rush the breath and your heart beats faster than usual, stop and start breathing deeply through both of your nostrils. Once you find your composure back, try again with 4-6 counts.

4. THE 4-2-6 BREATH (BREATHING WITH RETENTION/KUMBHAKA)

Scan the QR code or visit this URL to watch the video pose: https://balancedlivingbooks. com/chair-yoga-video-04/

SCAN ME

INSTRUCTIONS

1. Position your fingers in the same way with the anuloma viloma technique.
2. Start by deeply inhaling from your right nostril for four counts.
3. Press both nostrils with your thumb and ring finger. Hold your breath for two counts.
4. Release your ring finger while still closing your right nostril. Exhale from left nostril slowly for six counts.
5. Repeat the movements alternately for at least two minutes.

GENERAL TIPS

1. Increase the intensity once you get used to the 4-2-6 rhythm. Do it gradually, from 6-4-8, 8-6-10, and so on.

5. CLEANSING BREATH (KAPALBHATI)

Scan the QR code or visit this URL to watch the video pose: https://balancedlivingbooks. com/chair-yoga-video-05

SCAN ME

INSTRUCTIONS

1. Start with deep abdominal breathing a few times.
2. Inhale deeply and feel your belly expands.
3. As you exhale, do it hard as if you were forcing the air to out quickly. When doing this, you are supposed to feel that your belly button is drawn to the spine and your chest is slightly constricted to balance the squeeze coming from the abs.
4. After every exhalation, bring your body to a relax state in order to inhale slowly and deeply.
5. Repeat this pranayama for 8 to 20 times.

GENERAL TIPS

1. Do so without twitching your eyes or tightening your facial muscles.
2. There is no precise guideline on where you should place your hands. However, instead of placing them on your lap, touching your lower abdomen will make you more aware of your breathing and the pumping motion coming from the area between your pelvis and navel, as this is where air is being expelled.
3. Despite the forceful exhale, keep the inhalation like your usual breath.
4. Only practice this technique when your stomach is empty.

6. RAPID BREATHING (BHASTRIKA)

Scan the QR code or visit this URL to watch the video pose: https://balancedlivingbooks.com/chair-yoga-video-06/

INSTRUCTIONS

1. Do at least three to four repetitions of deep and calm breathing before beginning bhastrika.

2. After one deep breath, begin bhastrika by pushing a rapid and strong exhale. Quickly follow that with equally strong and fast inhalation and exhalation.

3. You can continue doing this breathing cycle for as long as you can. Once you feel as if you're running out of breath, take a break and go back to your normal breathing. If you're up to it, you can start the following round whenever you're ready.

COMMON MISTAKES TO AVOID

1. Despite the intense breathing, you shouldn't start to shake throughout your entire body. Only your abdomen, chest, and shoulders should move; the rest should stay at ease.

2. Attempt to maintain your torso's alignment. The vigorous breath shouldn't curve your spine.

GENERAL TIPS

1. Like kapalbhati pranayama, only practice this technique when your stomach is empty.

2. If you have a history of hypertension or vertigo, it isn't recommended to do this practice.

3. It's natural to notice that both your inhale and exhale only come to your chest, not deeper to your abdomen, due to its rapid tempo and vigorous breathing. There is no pausing or relaxation in the middle of the breath. However, you can stop whenever you feel fatigue or discomfort.

1. MOUNTAIN POSE

Scan the QR code or visit this URL to watch the video pose: https://balancedlivingbooks.com/chair-yoga-video-07/

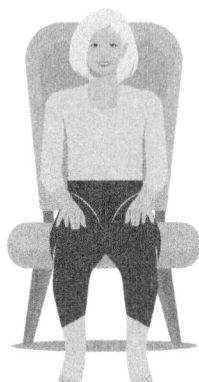

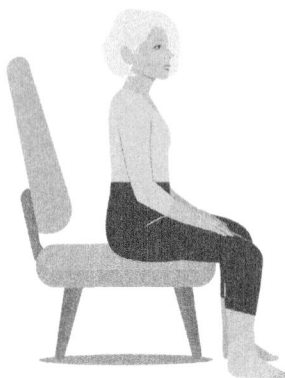

SCAN ME

INSTRUCTIONS

1. Sit in the center of your chair. Make sure your upper body feels comfortable without leaning to the back of the chair.
2. Keep your firm foundation by sitting on your sit bones. You can slide your butt slightly to the outer side, so your bottom can be steadier to bear your body weight.
3. Put your hands on your lap while maintaining your torso straight. Tuck your tailbone in and slightly pull your belly button toward your spine.
4. Keep your shoulders and neck muscles relaxed, with face to the front.
5. You can slightly roll your shoulders back to open your chest. Pull down your shoulder blades to help you be more comfortable and keep your spine properly aligned.
6. Spread your feet hip-width apart and position your heels in line with your knees.

COMMON MISTAKES TO AVOID

As the most basic pose, people often don't give much consideration about their postures when practicing mountain pose. In fact, since almost all poses start in this position, it will determine how safe your exercise is and whether you can reap the maximum benefits over the next sequence. For this reason, knowing some of the most common mistakes will help you to be more aware of your alignment and self-correct the pose if needed.

1. The spine curved backward.
2. The chest is too puffed out, leading to the spine arched forward.
3. Tense shoulders and neck, which can be seen from how close your ears are to your shoulders.
4. Using the flesh of your bottom as the foundation of your sitting instead of the sit bones.
5. The feet are too close or too far to the chair; making them not linear with the knees. This can affect the distribution of your body weight and make it uncomfortable to practice any movement.

GENERAL TIPS

1. It may be difficult to feel whether your spine is straight if your posture has been habitually slouched. One of the tips you can apply is to place the tips of your fingers slightly behind your buttocks. When you extend your elbows, your torso will automatically straighten. Initially, you might feel like your body is leaning too far back; however, over time, your body will get used to this better posture.

MODIFICATIONS AND VARIATIONS

1. If sitting on top of your sit bones hurts, you can add something to cushion your sit bone for more support, for example, by using a bolster or blanket. However, to make sure that your body weight can be proportionally distributed, choose the ones that aren't too thick or too soft. This will enable you to feel your sit bones actively gripping the padding.

VARIATION #1
INSTRUCTIONS

1. Clasp your fingers and push gently to your jaw so you can gaze at the ceiling.

2. Release the fingers. Move your hands to the back of your head and push it gently to draw your chin closer to your chest.

VARIATION #2
INSTRUCTIONS

1. Go back to the mountain pose. Raise your right arm to the ceiling.

2. Tilt your head to the right side and grab your left ear with your right hand. At the same time, straighten your left arm next to your left thigh until you feel a stretch in your left side of the neck.

3. Repeat the tilting of the head to the left side.

VARIATION #3
INSTRUCTIONS

1. In the mountain pose, bow your head.

2. Rotate the head 360 degrees slowly to the left. Do this twice, then repeat in the opposite direction.

Scan the QR code or visit this URL to watch the video pose: https://balancedlivingbooks.com/chair-yoga-video-08/

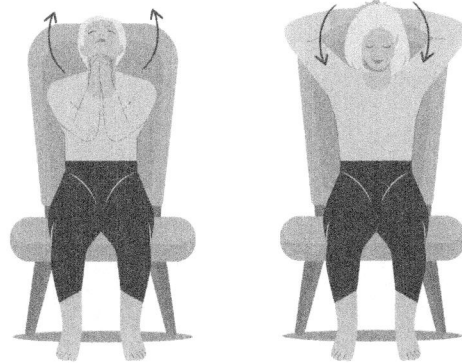

SCAN ME

Scan the QR code or visit this URL to watch the video pose: https://balancedlivingbooks.com/chair-yoga-video-09/

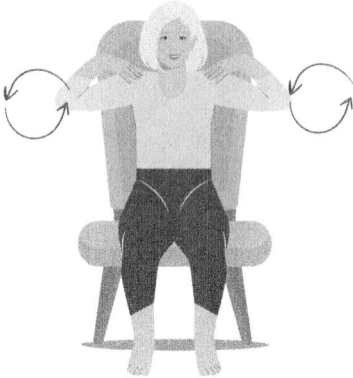

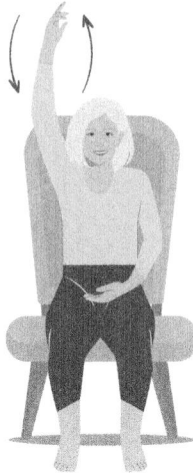

SCAN ME

VARIATION #1
INSTRUCTIONS

1. From the mountain pose, reach the shoulder with the fingers.
2. Open your elbows to the sides of your body to form 90-degree angle with your waist.
3. Make circular moves upward and downward at the shoulder hinges. Repeat several cycles, then do the same movement in the opposite direction.
4. Go back to the mountain pose. Extend your right arm to the ceiling.
5. Move your hands forward and then backward until they form a big loop. Repeat several cycles, then do the same movement in the opposite direction and with the left arm.

COMMON MISTAKES TO AVOID

1. When done too quickly, it is likely that only the arm muscles that move, not the joints in the shoulder area. So, take it slow and feel the stretch in the shoulder area.
2. Sometimes, focusing on your shoulders and arms' movement may cause your spine to unintentionally slouch backward. Make sure that your back is always aligned and your foundation remains steady.

VARIATION #2
INSTRUCTIONS

1. Prepare a strap, resistant band, a towel, or a belt.
2. Extend your arms in front of your chest while holding the strap.
3. Pull the strap to both sides while keeping your elbows straightened. Your hands should be opened way much wider than your shoulder-width.
4. Still keeping your arms actively engaged, move the strap upward above your head, then backward behind your back. Draw your hands further if you feel the pain. Focus on elongating your arms and the stretch around your shoulders, upper and lateral back.
5. Raise your arms again toward above the head, lower them forward to the chest, and repeat several times.

GENERAL TIPS

1. Make sure the strap is always tightly stretched. Adjust your hand grip when you notice the strap is loosened.
2. For starter, you can draw your hands wide opened. However, if you don't feel the stretch around the targeted muscles, narrow down the gap. The goal is to be able move your arms easily without pain while still experiencing the nice stretch.

VARIATION #1
INSTRUCTIONS

1. Extend your arms in front of your chest with all your fingers pointing forward.
2. Rotate your wrist inward (forming a circular motion) while the fingers make a squeezing motion. Do this for a few rounds, then repeat by rotating outwards.

VARIATION #2
INSTRUCTIONS

1. Go back to the mountain pose. Put your hands together right in front of your chest like a praying pose.
2. Press your palms lightly against each other. Stay there for at least five breaths and release.
3. Point your palms down until you can press the backs of your hands. Feel the stretch around the wrists and knuckles. Stay there for five breaths before going back to mountain pose.

Scan the QR code or visit this URL to watch the video pose: https://balancedlivingbooks.com/chair-yoga-video-10

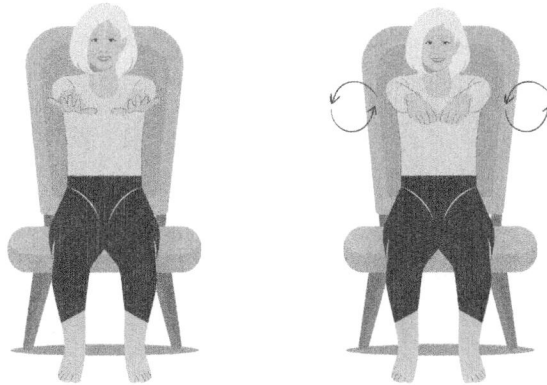

SCAN ME

VARIATION #3
INSTRUCTIONS

1. Take a deep breath and raise your arms.
2. Clasp your fingers and rotate your wrist outward so your palms are facing the ceiling.
3. Elongate your spine until you feel the pleasant stretch around your back, arms, and wrist.

VARIATION #4
INSTRUCTIONS

1. From the mountain pose, extend your arms in front of your chest with your hands facing each other without touching.
2. Bring your right hand to the outside of your left hand so that your hands are on top of each other.
3. Rotate your shoulder hinges externally, so your palms can clasp each other without lowering the position of your arms.
4. Drag your wrists toward your chest and insert them to the gap on your upper arms.
5. Extend your arms forward. Feel the stretch around all your wrists and lower arms. Stay there for a while, release and go back to a neutral position.
6. Repeat the same steps with your left hand on the outer side of your right hand.

COMMON MISTAKES TO AVOID

1. When rotating the wrist, don't just move your lower arms; instead, engage all the muscles from the elbow up to the shoulders.
2. Always keep your fingers active when pressing the palms.

Scan the QR code or visit this URL to watch the video pose: https://balancedlivingbooks.com/chair-yoga-video-11

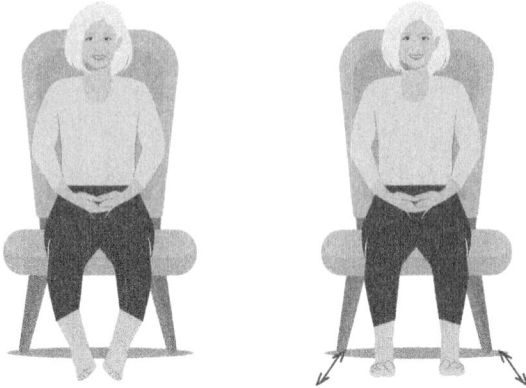

SCAN ME

INSTRUCTIONS

1. From the mountain pose, tilt the inner side of your feet so your soles rest only on the outer edge. Press gently for several seconds before going back to the initial position.

2. Tilt the heels and rest your feet on the balls of your toes. You can sway them back and forth and side by side, as if you were giving a gentle massage to those balls. After holding that position for several seconds, rest the soles by positioning them back on the floor.

3. Put pressure on your heels, firmly but gently. Flex your toes upward, then tuck them in beneath your forefoot.

4. Apply slight pressure until a stretch is felt in the joints and muscles of the toes. In this point, you can lift your heels to deepen the stretch.

GENERAL TIPS

Although experiencing and hearing the sounds of cracked knuckles is common during this sequence, it doesn't mean that should be our focus. Don't force or allocate too much body weight just to "pop" them. The pressure should be just enough to stimulate the nerves and muscles.

POSES OR ASANA

1. MODIFIED CAT-AND-COW (MARJARYASANA-BITILASANA)

INSTRUCTIONS

1. Elongate your arms to the ceiling.

2. Inhale and bring your arms slightly behind your head. Let your back arch and your chest open.

3. Exhale and draw your arms to the front of your chest while curving your spine. In this position, your chest must be drawn closer to the chest without raising your shoulders toward the ears.

4. Repeat for several cycles.

Scan the QR code or visit this URL to watch the video pose: https://balancedlivingbooks.com/chair-yoga-video-12

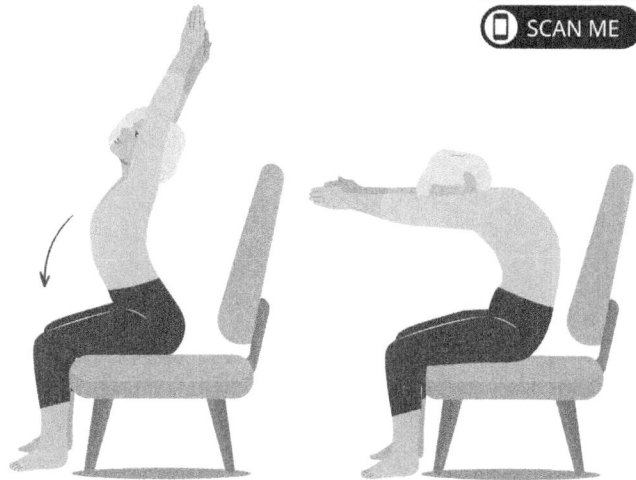

COMMON MISTAKES TO AVOID

1. Instead of just tucking your abdomen in and out, you should be able to feel the movement throughout each vertebra—from the lower back to the one right below your neck. You can monitor this by paying attention to your chest, shoulder blades, and hips. If you can sense the stretch in all those areas, then you are doing it right.

GENERAL TIPS

1. When arching your back, you can direct your gaze to the ceiling. However, only do this if you don't feel any dizziness or nausea. You can still look forward while focusing only on the movements of the spine.

MODIFICATIONS AND VARIATIONS

1. If elongating your arms while arching and rounding your back feels too heavy, we can modify this stretching. From mountain pose, you can directly arch and curve your spine without moving your hands' position. Press gently on your thighs or knees to help you stretch your torso.

Scan the QR code or visit this URL to watch the video pose: https://balancedlivingbooks.com/chair-yoga-video-13

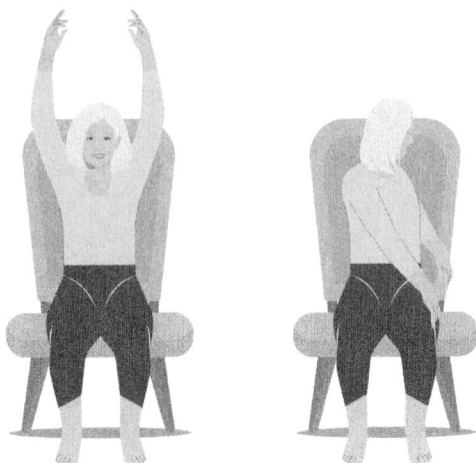

SCAN ME

INSTRUCTIONS

1. Raise your arms next to your ears.

2. Lower your right arm and grab your left knee. If comfortable, you can put your left hand on the backrest while the right hand gently presses the left knee. Feel the sensation as your spine is stretched and your right side of your torso is twisted gently.

3. Stay in this position for five breaths before repeating it in the opposite direction.

COMMON MISTAKES TO AVOID

1. Tensing your shoulders and neck when pressing the knee with your opposite hand. Keep them relaxed as we focus on the spine.

2. The sit bones are displaced; most likely, one side tilts as you twist your back. Hold your foundation firm.

3. Directly twist your back without raising your hands to the ceiling. This may seem trivial, but actually, the elongation serves a specific purpose. It helps to elongate all muscles around your back so you can twist more optimally.

GENERAL TIPS

1. You can direct your gaze backward to help your spine twist maximally. Alternatively, you can face sideways or anywhere that feels comfortable.

2. Don't move your hips and sitting position; but also, don't just move your rib cage. The twist should be from your waist upward.

MODIFICATIONS AND VARIATIONS

1. If comfortable, you can use both hands to grab the backrest of the chair. Slightly bend your elbows and deepen the twist to maximize the sensation of stretching.

2. While still twisting, you can opt to spread both hands as wide as possible. You may be unable to twist deeply, and that is alright as we combine core muscle exercise to maintain stability.

INSTRUCTIONS

1. From the mountain pose, take a deep breath as you extend both arms toward the ceiling. You can either clasp your fingers or just actively point them upward.

2. Exhale slowly as you bend your torso to the right side.

3. Lower your right arm while your left arm is still stretched next to your left ear.

4. Stay there for five breaths before returning to the initial position. Repeat with the opposite direction.

COMMON MISTAKES TO AVOID

1. Keep your chest open. Sometimes, people will unintentionally drag their chest and upper shoulder downward when bending their torso sideways. This isn't just leading to a "close chest," but also a possible rounded spine and tense shoulder blades—which negates the purpose of this pose in the first place.

2. Don't just bend your upper back. Instead, move your lower back and hips. This difference allows you to get the benefits more optimally.

GENERAL TIPS

1. When lowering one arm, imagine if you were trying to grab something on the floor without tilting your bottom. This will deepen the stretch around your outer side of bent torso.

2. Always pull down your shoulders; don't let them come too close to the ears.

MODIFICATIONS AND VARIATIONS

1. If you prefer to clasp your fingers, you can bend without releasing your arms. Strengthen your abs, as this variation relies on your core power to stabilize the upper body.

Scan the QR code or visit this URL to watch the video pose: https://balancedlivingbooks.com/chair-yoga-video-14

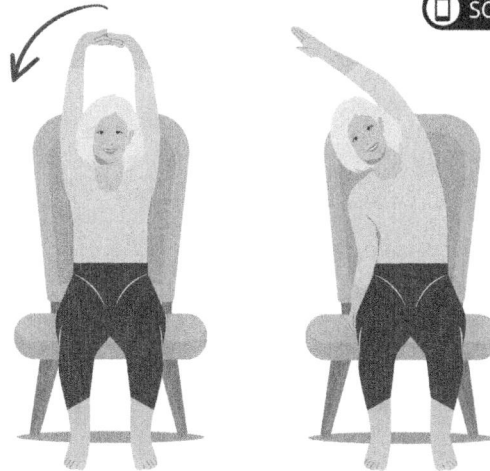

SCAN ME

Scan the QR code or visit this URL to watch the video pose: https://balancedlivingbooks.com/chair-yoga-video-15

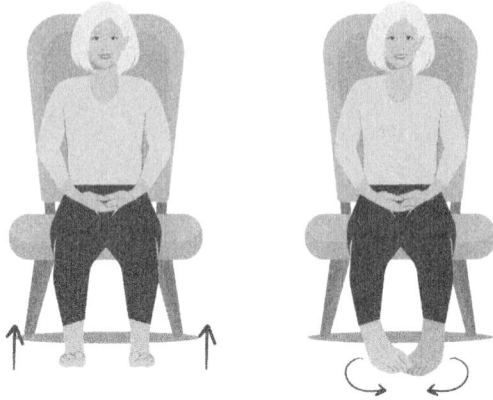

SCAN ME

INSTRUCTIONS

1. Lift both of your legs slightly away from the floor.
2. Make a circular motion so your ankle can feel the stretch.
3. While doing it, you can squeeze your toes to stimulate the muscles and nerves around the soles.
4. Repeat to the opposite direction.

COMMON MISTAKES TO AVOID

1. This practice targets the joints on your ankles and toes. Therefore, don't just randomly move your upper and lower legs; pay more attention on whether you feel the stretch around your soles and ankles.

MODIFICATIONS AND VARIATIONS

1. If lifting legs feels too heavy, you can try a milder variation. From the mountain pose, move your right leg a step forward without moving your sitting. After that, flex the sole of your foot until it rests on your heel. Pause for a few seconds, then continue by pointing your foot until stretching is felt in the instep area. You can rotate your ankle while still resting on the floor. Repeat the same procedure with the opposite foot.

INSTRUCTIONS

1. From the mountain pose, lift both your legs simultaneously so your soles float from the floor.
Maintain the bent knees to form 90 degrees.

2. Flex your soles and keep your toes active. Keep
your quadriceps engaged.

3. Pause for five breaths, then release, and repeat
for several times.

COMMON MISTAKES TO AVOID

1. Distribute your body weight proportionally
through the entire legs. Don't just engage your
thighs; but your calves and feet too.

2. There are no exact rules on how high you should
lift your legs. If this is your first, simply raise it slightly until the entire side of the sole of the foot
is floating from the floor. Over time, you will be
able to raise it higher without changing your
torso posture.

GENERAL TIPS

1. You can use a strap to help raise your legs and deepen the stretch around your quadriceps
and hamstrings.

Scan the QR code or visit this
URL to watch the video pose:
https://balancedlivingbooks.
com/chair-yoga-video-16

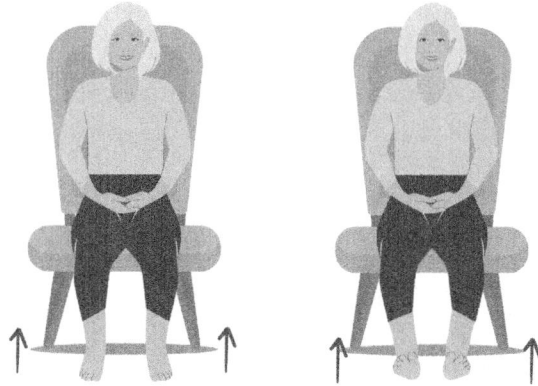

SCAN ME

6. QUADRICEPS AND HAMSTRINGS STRETCHING

Scan the QR code or visit this URL to watch the video pose: https://balancedlivingbooks.com/chair-yoga-video-17

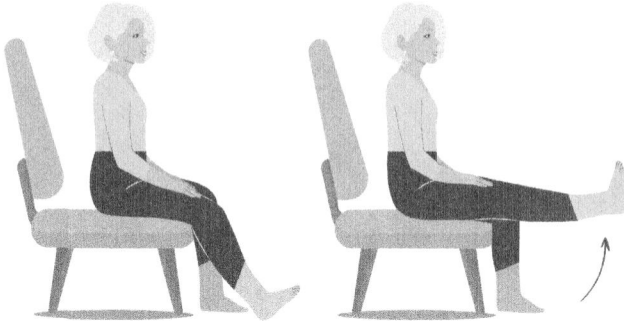

SCAN ME

INSTRUCTIONS

1. From the mountain pose, lift and straighten the right knee for a few seconds, then lower and straighten it again continuously. Do this for a minute, then go back to the neutral position.

2. Repeat the same movement for the left knee with the same time span.

GENERAL TIPS

1. When lifting your legs, your hands can grab the outer side of the chair to ensure that your bottom is still firmly grounded. Attempt not to lift your sit bones during the practice.

MODIFICATIONS AND VARIATIONS

1. For stiff hamstrings and quadriceps, we can modify this pose without lifting. The steps are as follows:

2. From the mountain pose, extend one leg forward so the knee is straightened.

3. Only your heel should touch the ground when you lift your toes. Keep your sole engaged.

4. As you inhale deeply, raise your arms high.

5. Exhale slowly and bend your torso upward. Aim to reach your flexed feet, but you can position your hand wherever you feel comfortable (on top of the thigh, on the knee, on the calf, or on the ankle). Feel the good stretch around your hamstring.

6. Inhale and lift your torso. Repeat this movement several times before moving to other leg.

7. To increase the intensity, you can repeatedly bend and straighten your legs several times without lowering them.

INSTRUCTIONS

1. Put a yoga block as your footstep for both feet. Alternatively, you can use a stack of books 4-9 inches high. You can also use towels or blankets that are folded several times so that they are firm enough to support your feet.

2. Bring the soles of the feet together and drop the knees to the outer sides.

3. Use your hands to apply gentle pressure on the knees. Feel your hips open as you maintain the position of your feet.

GENERAL TIPS

1. The placement of the block can be adjusted based on your hip's flexibility. The higher the block, the more open your hip feels.

2. You can also swing your legs up and down as if you were flapping the wings of a butterfly. This movement is useful for stimulating flexibility while opening the pelvis.

Scan the QR code or visit this URL to watch the video pose: https://balancedlivingbooks. com/chair-yoga-video-18

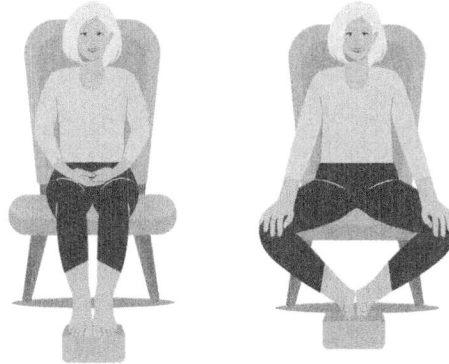

SCAN ME

Scan the QR code or visit this URL to watch the video pose: https://balancedlivingbooks. com/chair-yoga-video-19

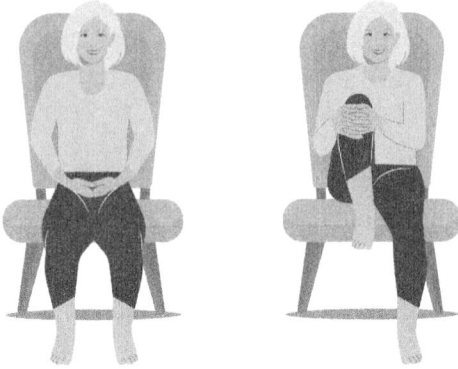

INSTRUCTIONS

1. From the mountain pose, drag one of your knees slowly toward your chest.

2. Use both hands to grab that bent leg and stay balanced.

3. Stay there for at least five breaths before lowering down your leg slowly back to the mountain pose.

4. Repeat the process with the opposite knee.

COMMON MISTAKES TO AVOID

1. Avoid leaning your back to the backrest while dragging your knees closer to the chest. Maintain the position of your torso by only moving your lower limbs.

2. Neither your bottom nor your shoulder should be tilted.

INSTRUCTIONS

1. From the mountain pose, bring your hands behind your lower back and interlace the fingers tightly.

2. Once your fingers are locked securely, straighten the elbows. Feel the stretch on your arms and shoulder blades. Keep gazing upward as you draw your chest higher, facing the ceiling.

3. You can add the sequence by bending your torso and uplifting your arms without releasing your interlocked fingers to deepen the stretch.

COMMON MISTAKES TO AVOID

1. While interlacing your fingers tightly can help you elongate and uplift your arms, doing it too tightly wouldn't make the pose any better. The grip should be firm, but make sure the elbow's joints can still move freely. Activate the muscles on your upper arms and scapula while opening your chest further to move your hands easily.

Scan the QR code or visit this URL to watch the video pose: https://balancedlivingbooks.com/chair-yoga-video-20

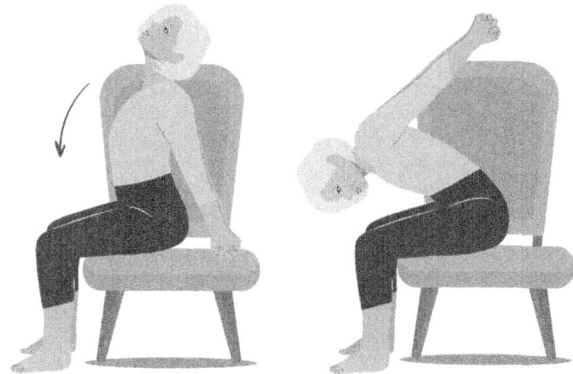

MODIFICATIONS AND VARIATIONS

1. Aside from interlocked fingers, there are some variations for this pose that you can follow up:

2. From the mountain pose, raise your right hand to the ceiling and tap your upper back. Then, bring your left hand to the back to hold your right arm. You can use a strap or belt if your hands can't reach each other. Do it for both sidevVvs with the same time span.

3. Bring your palms together in a namaste position, but do it on your back. This will not only open your chest but also stretch the wrists and lower arms. Keep in mind open your elbows outwardly to open the scapula and help your hands to reach each other easily.

4. Focus on the chest opening, not just how high you can lift your arms. If it feels too uncomfortable, you are allowed to modify the pose by not lifting your hands but dragging your scapula further to the back.

10. SEATED EAGLE POSE (GARUDASANA)

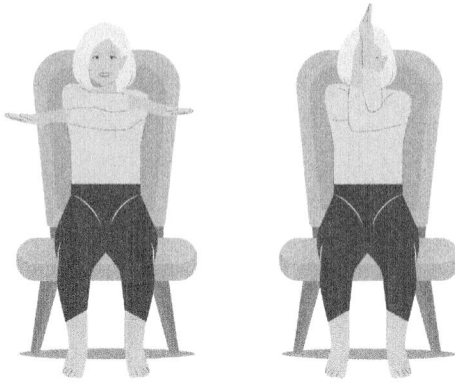

INSTRUCTIONS

1. From the mountain pose, stretch your arms in front of your chest.
2. Bend your elbows with your fingers pointing upward. Your lower arms should be upright with the upper arms.
3. Stack your right elbow on top of your left. The positions of your hands should naturally cross each other.
4. Interlace both fingers. Since the height is different, it's okay if your right hand can only grab the tips of the left fingers.
5. Inhale deeply and slightly lift both elbows until your upper arms are perpendicular toward your chest. You can push your shoulders slightly forward until you feel a nice pull in your scapula.
6. Exhale slowly while releasing your torso back to neutral alignment.
7. Release the wrapped arms, and repeat with the left arm on top of the right.

MODIFICATIONS AND VARIATIONS

1. If comfortable, you can add variation with back bending. Do this step-by-step to practice:
2. As you take a deep breath, arch your spine and face toward the ceiling while raise your arms higher. The position of upper and lower arms shouldn't be changed to maintain their parallel alignment. The more arched the back, the higher the hand position and the more the scapula is pushed forward.
3. When exhaling, bend forward your spine and draw your elbows closer to your belly button.
4. Tuck your belly in and lower your gaze. You can practice this advanced variation several times.

11. SEATED FORWARD BEND (PASCHIMOTTANASANA)

INSTRUCTIONS

1. From the mountain pose, position both feet slightly wider than the hips, approximately one step each to the left and right.

2. Inhale deeply as you elongate your spine by extending your arms to the ceiling. You can position your fingers either by clasping or clenching them into a fist.

3. Exhale slowly as you start bending your lower waist forward. Drop your abdomen between your inner thighs. Your face should be in a relaxed state while you rest your shoulders around the knees.

4. Hug your shins with both hands. Alternatively, keep your arms stretched forward while maintaining spine's alignment.

5. Stay there for at least five breaths.

6. To go back to the initial position, raise your torso slowly while keep activating both arms.

Scan the QR code or visit this URL to watch the video pose: https://balancedlivingbooks.com/chair-yoga-video-22

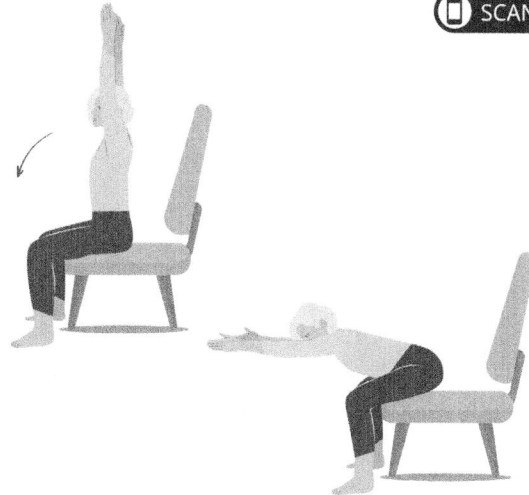

SCAN ME

COMMON MISTAKES TO AVOID

1. Bending the upper back instead of lower waist. Also, only bend as far as you feel comfortable, even if it's just a slight move.

GENERAL TIPS

1. Always squeeze your abdomen, especially when elongating your torso back to the mountain pose.

2. Instead of putting pressure on your back, give more power to your belly and arms in order to bend and lift easily.

3. Clasp or squeeze your fingers harder to help your back keep elongated when bending and lifting.

MODIFICATIONS AND VARIATIONS

1. You can add a further modification by opening your hips widely toward the outer side of your chair. Your sitting position should be slightly closer to the back of the chair so that there is enough space between your inner thighs. Bend your torso until your abdomen touches the chair. Feels the deep stretch around your hips and lower back.

2. After that, drag your arms under the seat through the space between your inner thighs. Keep your elbows stretched and straightened with fingertips touching the floor.

12. SEATED FORWARD BEND WITH TWO CHAIRS

Scan the QR code or visit this URL to watch the video pose: https://balancedlivingbooks.com/chair-yoga-video-23

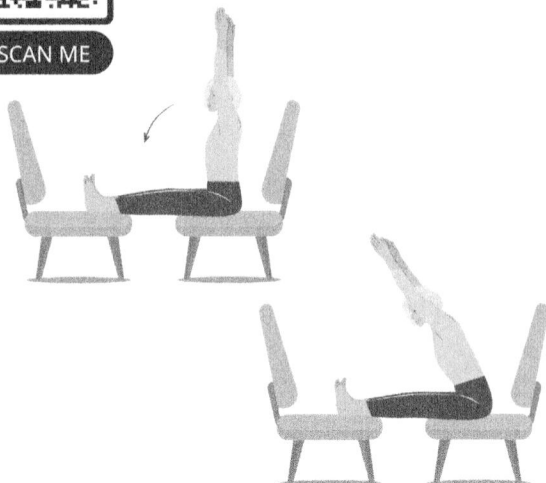

SCAN ME

INSTRUCTIONS

1. Prepare two chairs with the same height. Position them facing each other, roughly the length of your legs.

2. Sit on one chair and put your legs on the other. Make sure your knees can be fully extended and the soles of your feet stay on the seat, not protruding backwards.

3. Keep your feet actively engaged with toes pointing upward.

4. Take a deep breath and extend your hands.

5. As you exhale, bend your elongated spine forward. Rest your lower belly on your upper thigh and be mindful with your alignment.

6. Depending on your flexibility levels, you can put your hands on your thighs, knees, ankles, or soles—wherever—without curving your spine. Other options, you can grab the side edges of the spare chair if you feel that doing so will make the foundation steadier.

13. SEATED CHILD POSE (ADHO MUKHA VIRASANA)

INSTRUCTIONS

1. Prepare two chairs; one for you to sit, and the other is to rest your hands while bending your torso forward. This spare chair can be made more comfortable by placing a blanket or small pillow on it.

2. From the mountain pose, take a deep breath while raising your hands upward to lengthen your spine.

3. Exhale slowly and bend your torso forward. Put your head on the pillow or the extra chair. Let your hands rest comfortable next to your head; either on the seat or on top of the backrest.

4. Stay as long as you need.

GENERAL TIPS

1. Although this pose is perfect for resting, catching up breathing rhythm, or wrapping up your exercise session, it's best to keep your elbow engaged and the spine stretched.

Scan the QR code or visit this URL to watch the video pose: https://balancedlivingbooks.com/chair-yoga-video-24

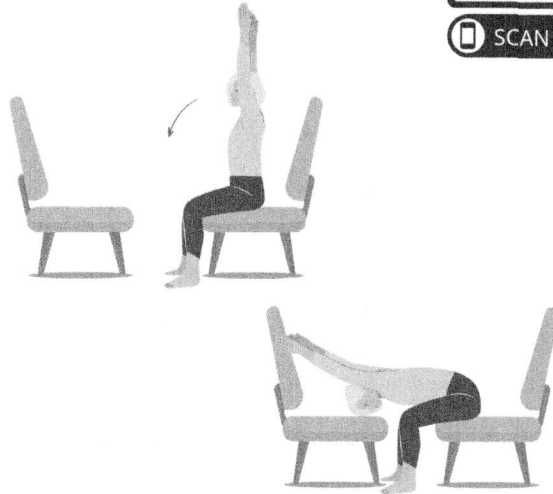

14. MODIFIED DOWNWARD FACING DOG (ADHO MUKHA SVANASANA)

Scan the QR code or visit this URL to watch the video pose: https://balancedlivingbooks.com/chair-yoga-video-25

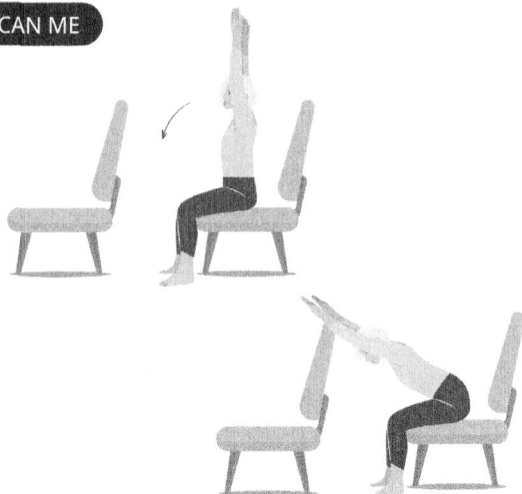

SCAN ME

INSTRUCTIONS

1. Using two chairs. position the spare one with the backrest facing you. The distance should be approximately the length of your legs.

2. From the mountain pose, take a deep breath and extend your arms upward.

3. As you exhale, reach the backrest of the spare chair with both your hands while straightening your back.

COMMON MISTAKES TO AVOID

1. No hollows in the upper back area. Push the scapula slightly upward so that your back and neck alignment is properly straightened.

2. There shouldn't be any cavity on the lower back. To avoid this, always tuck your tailbone in. You can slightly squeeze the glutes and abs as well.

GENERAL TIPS

1. To imitate the original pose, you may use the spare chair with shorter backrest. This will enable your body to have a slight inversion pose. However, if doing so can increase the risk of falling, then using the chair with same height or slightly higher. Just focus on your spine's posture and grip strength.

INSTRUCTIONS

1. From the mountain pose, elevate your arms as you inhale deeply.

2. Exhale slowly and start bending your torso into approximately 45 degrees.

3. Hold your position for five breaths, then release. Repeat several times in one session to train your core muscles.

COMMON MISTAKES TO AVOID

1. Don't simply bend your torso slightly. Make sure you can feel your abs squeezing and your spine straightened to keep you balanced.

2. Lowering your arms. When you are avoiding that, your abs will be more stimulated to balance your body weight as you move your hands higher.

3. Stepping your feet forward, regardless how light you feel around your core muscles. While it feels comfortable, unfortunately doing this will negate the goal of this sequence.

GENERAL TIPS

1. Although the name of this pose has consisted the word "chair" by itself, it doesn't mean that there is no point to modify it literally with chair. In fact, this can be a warm-up to strengthen core muscles before practicing other more challenging poses.

2. In bending position, make sure you have visual on your toes. If your knees prevent you from seeing your toes clearly, then you need to lower your torso position.

Scan the QR code or visit this URL to watch the video pose: https://balancedlivingbooks.com/chair-yoga-video-26

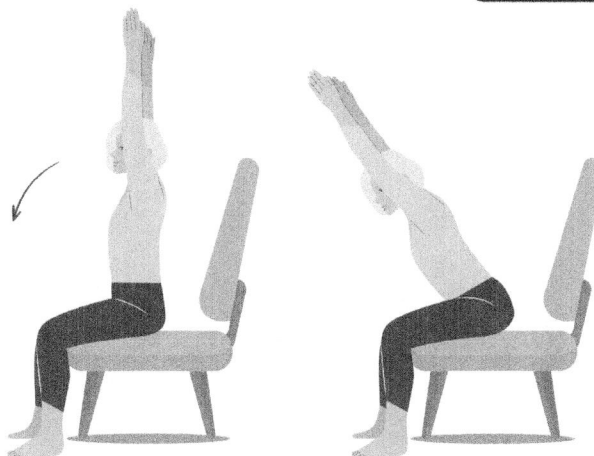

SCAN ME

Scan the QR code or visit this URL to watch the video pose: https://balancedlivingbooks. com/chair-yoga-video-27

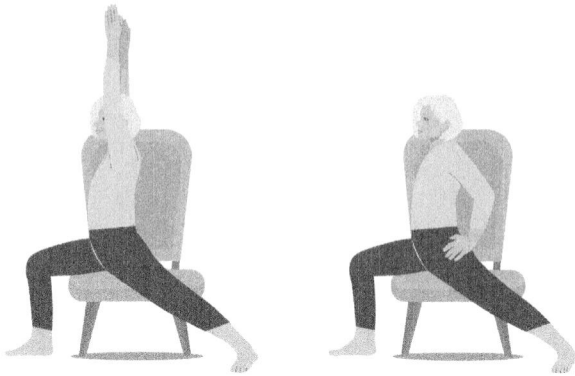

SCAN ME

INSTRUCTIONS

1. Sit on the side of your chair so the backrest is right next to your arm. Position your bottom on the rear edge of your sitting.
2. Bring your leg (that isn't blocked by the backrest) to the back of your body, as far as you feel comfortable to straighten the knee.
3. Your foot should be planted firmly with an angle of approximately 45 degrees outward. Don't lift your heels or fingers as you use this leg as a foundation.
4. Maintain the position of your forward leg, bent 90 degrees. Make sure your sole touches the floor firmly.
5. Raise your hands to the ceiling and straighten your elbows.
6. Hold for five breaths, then repeat to the opposite side.

COMMON MISTAKES TO AVOID

1. Your hips aren't square. This can be seen by whether your body is actually facing forward and perpendicular to the floor, or slightly moving to the side.
2. The back foot doesn't ground but stands on tiptoe. If you find it difficult to keep your footing, readjust your sitting position so that your back knee is straight but your heel is not lifted.

GENERAL TIPS

1. If it's difficult to position the pelvis straight ahead, you can slightly rest your body on the hip flexors of the back leg.
2. You can step on a block if your forward foot is unable to touch the floor completely.

17. SEATED WARRIOR II (VIRABHADRASANA II)

INSTRUCTIONS

1. From the Warrior I position, bring your torso sideways to the chair's backrest so that it is behind you.

2. Drop your arms so they are extended sideways, parallel to the ground.

3. To adjust the alignment of your arms and shoulders, start by positioning your palms to face the ceiling. Then, turn them upside down; but the rotation should be centered on your shoulder hinges.

4. Direct your gaze toward the tip of fingers that are parallel to the bent knee. That being said, if the right leg is bent, then face to the right side, and vice versa.

5. After holding for five breaths, release. Repeat to the opposite side.

Scan the QR code or visit this URL to watch the video pose: https://balancedlivingbooks.com/chair-yoga-video-28

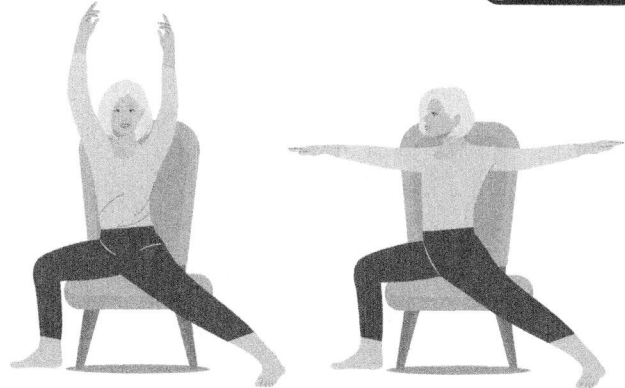

COMMON MISTAKES TO AVOID

1. When turning your palms to face the floor, don't just roll your lower arms. Make sure you feel the rotation up to the shoulder joints.

2. The inner side of the bent knee is slightly drawn forward in your body. Maintain the alignment until the bent knee forms a straight line with your ankle.

18. SEATED REVERSE WARRIOR / WARRIOR III

Scan the QR code or visit this URL to watch the video pose: https://balancedlivingbooks.com/chair-yoga-video-29

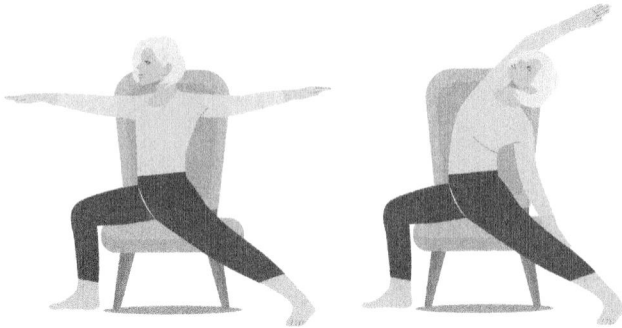

SCAN ME

INSTRUCTIONS

1. From Warrior II position, place one of your hands on the back of your thigh (where the knee is straightened), and the other hand is lifted to the ceiling.

2. Slowly lower your hand behind your thigh, as deep as you feel comfortable. Simultaneously, let your back arched and your chest is dragged higher and more open.

3. Maintain the position of your lifted arm to stay close to the ear.

4. Stay there for five breaths, then go back to neutral position before repeating the warrior sequences for the opposite side.

COMMON MISTAKES TO AVOID

1. Don't use your hand that is placed on the back of the thigh to solely support your arched back. Ideally, the body weight is always distributed properly between both legs. The gap between your shoulders and your ears can be an indicator; when it's to close, pull it down and strengthen your core.

2. Don't lock your elbow. Oftentimes, especially when the sequence gets heavier, people tend to hyperextend their joints. This can be seen in static alignment when the joint loses its full range of motion. Visually, it will be seen that your elbow is beyond 180 degrees as it out of alignment of the arm. Avoid this by maintaining balance and not forcing one point to load heavier weight than other body parts.

19. SEATED HUMBLE WARRIOR (BADDHA VIRABHADRASANA)

INSTRUCTIONS

1. From the Warrior I pose, stretch one leg sideways and straighten the knee.
2. Bring the opposite leg to the other side of the chair and bend it 90 degrees. Make sure both feet are planted firmly on the ground.
3. Put your hands on your waist.
4. Drag your torso next to your bent knee.
5. Stay there for five breaths, release, and repeat to the opposite direction.

COMMON MISTAKES TO AVOID

1. Don't resting your belly on your thigh. Avoid this by slightly moving your bent body away from the thigh (but don't too far) or keep it floating above your thigh. Tighten your abdominal muscles to keep your balance without resting anywhere.

GENERAL TIPS

1. If you practice this pose right after reverse warrior, all you need to do is bring your torso to the bent knee. Position one hand on your calf or ankle, and the other stretched up or to the side of your ear.

MODIFICATIONS AND VARIATIONS

1. To deeply open your rib cage and stretch your shoulders, you can interlock your fingers on the back, then straighten them upward as you bend your torso.

Scan the QR code or visit this URL to watch the video pose: https://balancedlivingbooks.com/chair-yoga-video-30

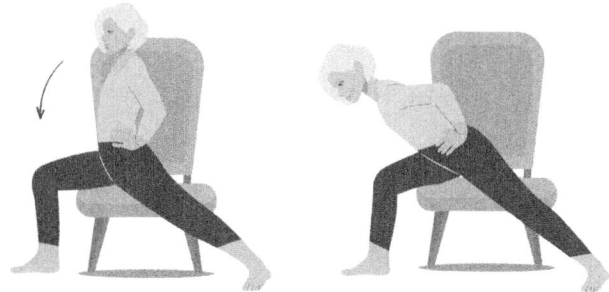

SCAN ME

20. MODIFIED EXTENDED SIDE ANGLE (UTTITA PARSVAKONASANA)

Scan the QR code or visit this URL to watch the video pose: https://balancedlivingbooks.com/chair-yoga-video-31

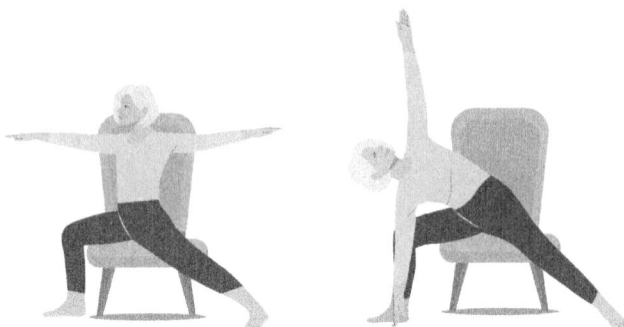

INSTRUCTIONS

1. Stretch one leg sideway and bend the other leg to the opposite direction to form a 90-degree angle. Put your hand on the ground, right next to your bent knee. Or, if you are already from the reverse warrior position, directly lower your lifted arm to reach the floor. Do this without moving your leg position.

2. Position your other hand in a ceiling-pointing position. If possible, you can drag this arm next to your ear without drawing your chest downward.

3. Stay there for five breaths and repeat to the opposite side.

GENERAL TIPS

1. It's easy to unintentionally drag your upward shoulder to the floor. To avoid this, imagine there is a big wall against your back. Attempt to press all side of your back to this wall. You can do this by slightly pushing the upward shoulder back (but not too much) and tuck your tailbone in.

MODIFICATIONS AND VARIATIONS

1. If reaching the floor feels too far, you can use a block for your hand to rest. The placement should be in the inner side of your midfoot, but the height can be adjusted based on your flexibility.

2. For a milder variation, you can rest your elbow on your thigh instead of reaching your hand to the floor. Keep your shoulders relaxed and rely on your core muscles to stay balanced.

21. MODIFIED EXTENDED TRIANGLE POSE (TRIKONASANA)

INSTRUCTIONS

1. Sit in the mountain pose with the chair facing forward.

2. Gently slide one of your legs sideway and straighten the knee. Keep your soles firmly planted on the floor.

3. Let the other leg facing forward with knee bent 90 degrees.

4. Take a deep breath and raise your arms.

5. Exhale and side-bend your torso. You can put your hand either on your extended knee, shin, thigh, ankle, or the floor. The lower you can reach, the deeper the stretch you feel in your side torso and hamstring.

6. For your other arm, you can adjust the placement based on your flexibility:

7. On your waist

8. Extended to the ceiling

9. Close to your ear

10. After holding for several breaths, go back to initial position slowly and repeat for the opposite side.

Scan the QR code or visit this URL to watch the video pose: https://balancedlivingbooks.com/chair-yoga-video-32

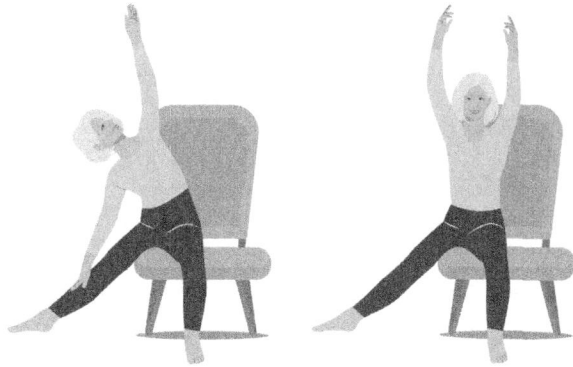

SCAN ME

COMMON MISTAKES TO AVOID

1. Your ribcage is a little inclined toward the floor. Bring your shoulder back so that your chest is open, but avoid opening it all the way so that your torso is out of alignment.

2. Tilting your bottom while extending the arm.

GENERAL TIPS

1. Regardless of your hand's position, make sure that your fingers, palms, and arms are actively engaged.

2. If your arm is extended upward, you can direct your gaze toward the tip of your fingers. But if your hand is on your waist, face forward in neutral position. It's recommended not to gaze downward since this is prone to curve your back and close your rib cage.

Scan the QR code or visit this URL to watch the video pose: https://balancedlivingbooks.com/chair-yoga-video-33

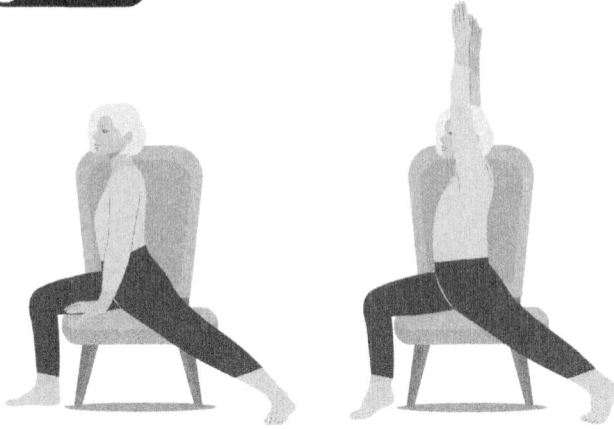

SCAN ME

INSTRUCTIONS

1. Sit on the side of your chair.

2. Straighten one of your feet backward. Raise the heel so that only the toes and balls of the foot are firmly planted on the floor.

3. With a deep inhale, bring your arms upward while still gazing forward.

4. Stay there for five breaths before releasing and repeating on the opposite direction.

COMMON MISTAKES TO AVOID

1. Don't just lift the heel slightly. Ideally, your heel and the balls of your foot are stacked in a straight line. Feel that all muscles around your foot are engaged and stretched.

GENERAL TIPS

1. Depending on the size and shape of your chair, it's most likely that sitting on the rear edge of the chair will make it easier for your leg to move backward and to bend your toes. In addition, this can also help your forward leg to form 90 degrees since the back of your knee is supported by the edge of the chair.

2. Step your foot further back if you find it difficult to straighten your knee or if you don't feel any stretch in your hamstring and calf areas.

3. If you feel any misalignment on your hips, slowly and gently stand up with the aid of your toes on your rear leg. However, if this feels overwhelming, you can start over to adjust your sitting and re-position your legs.

INSTRUCTIONS

1. Start by sitting in the mountain pose with your body facing forward (the backrest is behind your back).

2. Grab your right knee and drag it closer to your chest. Hug it as deeply as you feel comfortable.

3. Bring your feet to a horizontal position, so your knee is dropped toward the outer side. Position your hand grips on the knee and calf or ankle areas. Sway your leg (still in a horizontal position) inward and outward to open your pelvis further.

4. With full flexion from the hip joint, put your right ankle on your left lap. Attempt to maintain your lifted leg to stay in a straight line.

5. Take a deep breath and elevate your arms upward. Ensure your back is still in a proper alignment.

6. Exhale slowly and draw your torso forward. You can position your hands either to stay outstretched to the sides of your head or on put them on top of your bent knee and ankle to apply gentle pressure.

7. Stay on that position for a few seconds. Release and repeat to the left leg.

Scan the QR code or visit this URL to watch the video pose: https://balancedlivingbooks. com/chair-yoga-video-34

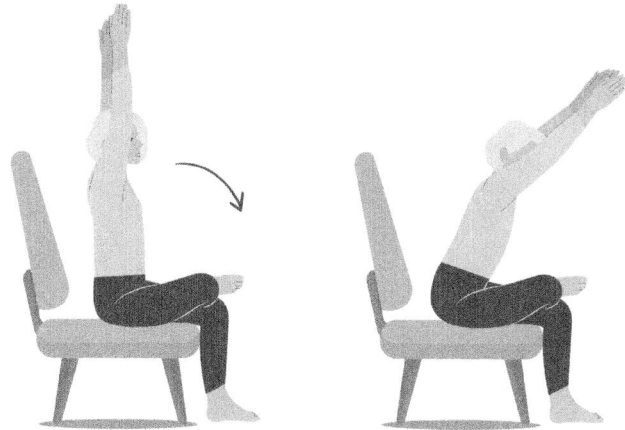

SCAN ME

24. WIDE-LEGGED SEATED FORWARD BEND (UPAVISTHA KONASANA)

Scan the QR code or visit this URL to watch the video pose: https://balancedlivingbooks.com/chair-yoga-video-35

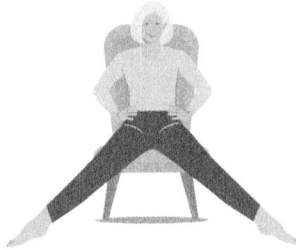

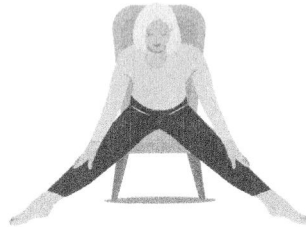

SCAN ME

INSTRUCTIONS

1. From the mountain pose, open your feet sideways so they are wider than hip-width.

2. Extend your legs and straighten your knees. Keep your feet pointing forward.

3. Take a deep breath and put your hands on your waist.

4. As you exhale, drop your chest forward without resting your belly on the seat or the thighs. Tone your abs to keep your spine aligned.

5. Bring your hands to grab your shins or calves.

MODIFICATIONS AND VARIATIONS

1. After grabbing your shins, you can put your hands on the middle front ground. Bend your elbows and deepen your forward bending. Give firm pressure to the floor using your hands to keep your body steady while tightening your core muscles.

2. Continue the previous modification by extending your arms below the chair, as far as you feel comfortable. Press your hands against the ground to lower your body. Keep all the muscles engaged.

3. If you feel that the stretch in the initial pose is too deep, you can ease the intensity by using two blocks. Instead of grabbing your shins or calves, put your palms on blocks that are positioned between your legs, next to your head. You don't have to bend your elbows and torso deeply, as long as the bend comes from the lower waist and your spine keep elongated all the time.

INSTRUCTIONS

1. Open your feet wide apart as you sit comfortable in the middle of the chair. Feel the stretch on the inner thighs and hips.

COMMON MISTAKES TO AVOID

1. Don't stand on tiptoe; instead, make sure both feet are planted firmly to the floor.
2. Don't just open your hands. Make sure your elbow is in a straight line with your chest and engage the muscle to keep them steady.

GENERAL TIPS

1. Use the hand movement as an opportunity to open your chest and tuck your tailbone in. When viewed from the side, your torso will look like a straight line.

MODIFICATIONS AND VARIATIONS

1. If you can maintain this position for five breaths without difficulty, you can follow with further variations.
2. From the goddess pose, clasp your fingers behind your head. Your elbows will naturally spread sideways.
3. Bend your torso to the right, at a 45 degrees angle. Use the muscles over your neck, shoulders, arms, and abs to maintain the position. Don't rest your elbows on your thighs, and keep your chest open.
4. Go back to the goddess pose and repeat this variation to the left side.
5. Here's another variation involving side bending and core strength:
6. From the goddess pose, rest your right elbow to your right thigh. Engage your hip flexors and glutes firmly so that your hips do not tilt, your shoulders do not strain, and your neck is at ease.
7. Extend your left arm next to your left ear.
8. Stay there for five breaths before releasing and repeating on the left side.
9. You can incorporate an extended side angle into this pose as well.
10. From the goddess pose, lower your right arm to touch either your right ankle or the floor. Use a yoga block if it feels too stiff to bend that deep.
11. Point your left hand straight up or next to your left ear.
12. Stay there for five breaths and repeat for the left side.
13. **The revolving goddess pose (*parivrtta utkata konasana*)** is a more advance variation that includes twisting. It's a great pose to release the strain on your shoulders and upper back.
14. From the goddess pose, drop your hands to your knees. Keep them engaged without slouching your back.
15. Bend your body forward without resting your belly on your inner thighs. Direct your gaze upward to the ceiling.
16. Bend your left elbow and simultaneously draw your chest toward your left thigh. Keep your right arm stretched. Feel the stretch around your waist as you twist your lower back.
17. Back to neutral position, then repeat to the right side.

Scan the QR code or visit this URL to watch the video pose: https://balancedlivingbooks.com/chair-yoga-video-36

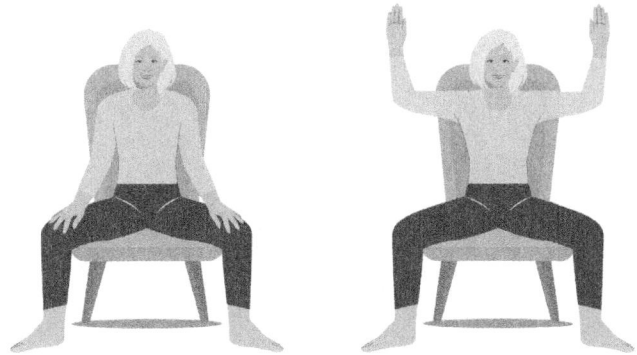

SCAN ME

Scan the QR code or visit this URL to watch the video pose: https://balancedlivingbooks.com/chair-yoga-video-37

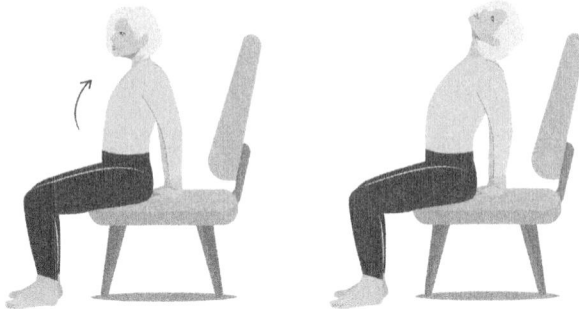

SCAN ME

INSTRUCTIONS

1. From the mountain pose, place your fingers slightly behind your bottom. If there is enough space, move your sitting forward to be closer to the edge of the chair.

2. Roll your shoulders to open your chest, and prepare your spine to curve. Position both elbows inward as if your upper arms are pinching your armpits.

3. Start curving your back forward and puffing your chest as far as you feel comfortable.

4. Keep the neck muscle relaxed by directing your gaze toward the ceiling. But if it doesn't feel comfortable, face forward without tensing your neck or shoulders.

5. Stay there for five breaths before returning to the neutral position.

COMMON MISTAKES TO AVOID

1. The elbow does not pinch inward, but instead opens outward.

2. Not changing the position of the footrest when sitting closer to the edge of the chair. As a result, knees and heels are not properly aligned.

GENERAL TIPS

1. Your hands can grab the outer or back edge below the backrest for more support, but if only the design of your chair allows you to do so.

MODIFICATIONS AND VARIATIONS

1. You can position your hands around your lower back with fingers pointing downward. Use your hands to gently push the lower back, and feel the pleasant sensation of stretching there.

INSTRUCTIONS

1. In th mountain pose, sit slightly closer to the front edge of the chair. Give enough space around your bottom to place your hands later.

2. Put the tips of your fingers behind your bottom.

3. While taking a deep breath, push the seat of the chair using your fingertips while simultaneously driving your chest upwards. Depending on how deep you want to bend backwards, pull your chin towards the ceiling.

4. Hold this posture for several seconds while taking five shallow breaths toward your rib cage.

COMMON MISTAKES TO AVOID

1. If you have glaucoma, refrain from performing this stance.

GENERAL TIPS

1. Do this sequence without straining your neck and shoulders. You can lessen the curving force of your backbend if it helps you feel more relaxed.

2. Depending on how the chair is built, you can rest your head on the backrest. The ideal position is either the top or the back of your head, but not the lower head. However, avoid applying pressure to your neck or head. Be mindful of how your body weight is distributed.

Scan the QR code or visit this URL to watch the video pose: https://balancedlivingbooks.com/chair-yoga-video-38

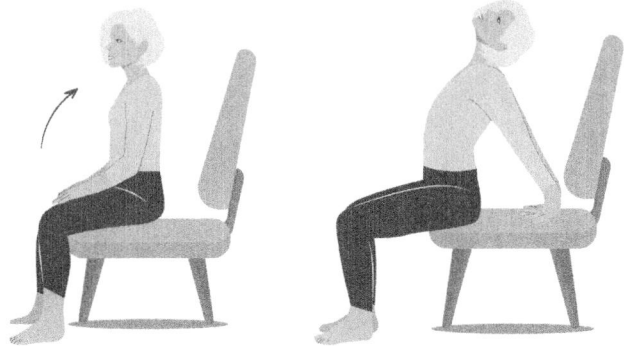

SCAN ME

SCAN ME

Scan the QR code or visit this URL to watch the video pose: https://balancedlivingbooks.com/chair-yoga-video-39

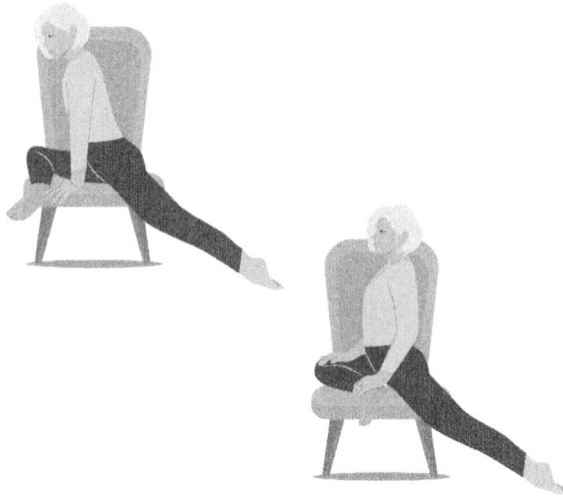

INSTRUCTIONS

1. Sit on the side of the chair so that the backrest is adjacent to your arm. If your chair seat is wide enough, make sure your sitting position is right next to the backrest, not in the middle.

2. Draw your feet that are at the outer edge of the chair (not the one that is blocked by the backrest) towards the back. Elongate the hamstrings by extending your knee.

3. Position the instep on the floor so that the sole of your rear foot is facing the ceiling.

4. Carefully bend your forward leg so your ankle and calf are on top of the chair seat. If there is no pain, attempt to position your ankle and knee in a straight line. Otherwise, you can drag your ankle closer to your hips. Either way, make sure to keep your hips stay square.

5. There are a few options for hands' placement:

6. Put your hands on the inner knee and ankle; give a slight pressure open the hip socket even deeper.

7. If there is available space next to your rear thigh, put your hand there. Push the chair gently to help your back be more aligning. Doing so will automatically deepen the stretch around your hamstrings, glutes, and hip flexors. The other hand can be placed either on your back of rear leg or the backrest.

COMMON MISTAKES TO AVOID

1. Tilting your bottom as you lift one leg. Ensure your hips are square throughout the entire sequence.

2. Let your belly rest on top of your bent leg. To avoid this, move forward closer to the edge of your knee, so there will be enough space between the calf and inner thigh for your belly.

3. Positioning your ankle near your belly when lifting it instead of ensuring their parallel alignment.

GENERAL TIPS

1. Compared to other modified pose using a chair, this may be categorized as one of upper intermediate ones. To ensure safety and comfortability, it's best to incorporate lots of warm-ups and stretching that target hamstrings and hip flexors. This precaution will ease the tense when crossing your legs.

2. After lifting your leg, you can stimulate flexibility by swaying your thighs up and down. To help your pelvis loosen up more, softly press down on the inside of your knee. Do this for a few seconds with several repetitions before continuing the sequence.

3. If it feels too overwhelming, you can stop once your ankle has been lifted to your lap. This pose itself is also beneficial to loosen your stiff pelvic; therefore, you can practice this even if you don't intend to complete the entire pigeon pose.

INSTRUCTIONS

1. Position your sitting slightly backward, almost reaching the backrest.

2. Grab your right knee with both hands and bring your foot (or only the heel if there is no enough space to rest your sole) to the seat.

3. Extend your left leg forward. Flex your toes and make sure your left heel is grounded firmly.

4. As you take a deep breath, elongate your spine.

5. Exhale and twist your lower back. Drag your left elbow to the outer side of your knee and your right hand toward the backrest. Use your hands to deepen the stretch.

6. Stay there for five breaths and extend your hands to the ceiling again as your torso goes back to neutral position.

7. Still bending the right knee, now twist your body to the right.

8. Put the back of your right elbow to the inner side of your knee. Simultaneously, grab the backrest with your left hand. Deepen the twist as far as you feel comfortable.

9. Go back to the initial position after pausing for five breaths. Start over in the opposite direction.

Scan the QR code or visit this URL to watch the video pose: https://balancedlivingbooks.com/chair-yoga-video-40

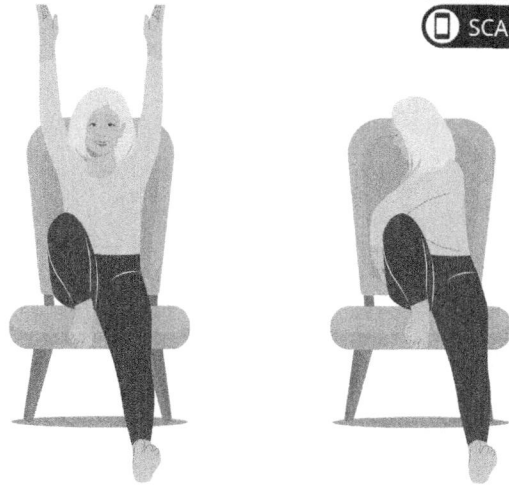

GENERAL TIPS

1. Aim your gaze to adjust the direction of the twisting. Make sure there is no strain around your neck and shoulders.

MODIFICATIONS AND VARIATIONS

1. If it feels too challenging to fully twist your lower back, it may be because you need something to make the buttock higher than the footrest. If that is the case, roll a towel, blanket, or pillow and place it beneath your bottom. However, make sure that this property isn't too high which may lead to unstable foundation.

30. MODIFIED BOAT POSE (NAVASANA)

Scan the QR code or visit this URL to watch the video pose: https://balancedlivingbooks.com/chair-yoga-video-41

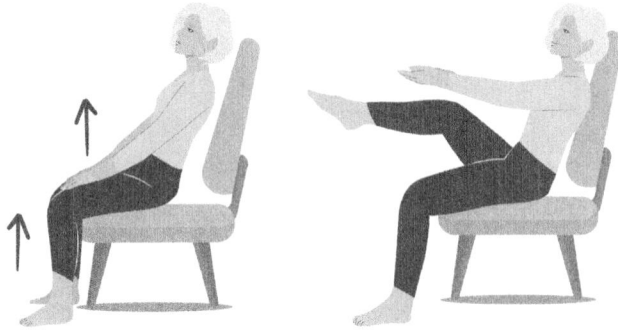

SCAN ME

INSTRUCTIONS

1. Sit a little bit closer to the front edge of the chair, but not so close that it increases the risk of falling. Provide enough space for your torso (in a straight position) to lean to form an angle of approximately 45 degrees.

2. Reach behind the right knee and bring it toward the chest without changing the position of the torso.

3. Keep the muscle on your lifted leg activated. Point your soles and toes.

4. Release your grip by extending your hands in front of your chest. Use your core muscles to keep the balance and gently squeeze your hamstring to maintain the alignment.

5. For more challenge, you can lift the other leg and attempt to balance your foundation. Alternatively, lower your lifted leg and repeat with the opposite side.

COMMON MISTAKES TO AVOID

1. Rounded back and tense shoulders.

2. The position of your calf is too close to the back of your thigh. Pull it upward, as far as you feel comfortable.

GENERAL TIPS

1. When lifting one leg, you can use a yoga block under the other leg to provide additional support.

2. Before trying to activate both legs simultaneously, it would be wise if you try to get used to balancing on lifting one leg first. Challenge yourself to uplift your lower leg until it is parallel to your knee and chest.

3. Another more advanced variation is extending your lifted leg forward without the help of your hands to keep the balance. Do this alternately, with several seconds of pauses for each movement.

Unlike other poses that start with a seated position on a chair, this move requires a chair only for leg support. Only do this pose if you can and are comfortable exercising in a reclining position. It's best to lie down on top of a non-slippery mat for safety and comfortability.

Scan the QR code or visit this URL to watch the video pose: https://balancedlivingbooks. com/chair-yoga-video-42

INSTRUCTIONS

1. In a lying position, position your hands at your sides with both palms touching the floor.

2. Elevate your legs on top of a chair. Make sure your feet are on the seat (not extending backward through the gap under the backrest or the side of the chair if you are lying on the sideways).

3. Position your feet against the seat, with the soles of your feet fully planted on the chair, not just the heels or balls of your feet.

4. Start lifting your hips with taking a deep breath. Elevate as higher as you feel comfortable. Stay there for several seconds.

5. When lowering your pelvic, do it slowly; vertebrae by vertebrae. Lower the vertebrae first at the top point you can lift, then further down to the buttocks.

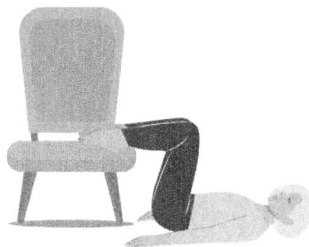

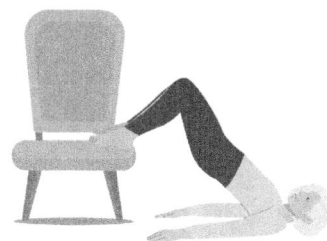

COMMON MISTAKES TO AVOID

1. Direct your focus and power on your hips and lower limbs. Don't bear weight in the neck or shoulder area. Keep the torso in a relaxed state.

2. Don't move your neck and head during elevating the hips—not even slightest. Gaze only at the ceiling, no need to turn your head in any direction.

3. Spreading your knees when lifting hips. Attempt to always keep your inner thighs against each other.

4. Lowering your hips from lower back first; worse, if you do it in a hurry.

GENERAL TIPS

1. When lifting your hips, grabbing the edge of your mattress can help you lift higher.

2. Keep your toes and soles active. The more engaged your feet, the steadier your footing that directly affect your lifting.

3. After releasing, make sure all vertebrae are touching the floor. Rock your back slowly as if you were massaging all sides of your back.

MODIFICATIONS AND VARIATIONS

To some extent, being aware of whether your inner thighs against each other while also focusing on elevating hips isn't always easy. We can overcome this by leveling up the intensity. Tuck a yoga block between your thighs. Pinch firmly as you lift your hips. By keeping the block from falling, you will always activate your inner thigh muscles.

32. SEATED TREE POSE (VRKSASANA)

Scan the QR code or visit this URL to watch the video pose: https://balancedlivingbooks.com/chair-yoga-video-43

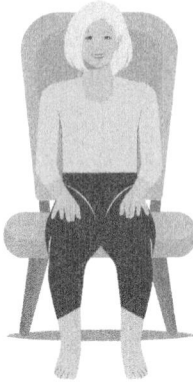

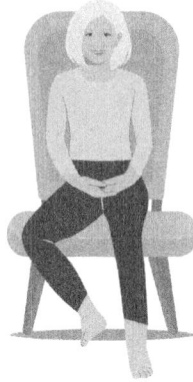

SCAN ME

INSTRUCTIONS

1. From the mountain pose, bring your position slightly to the front edge.
2. Straighten your left knee forward. Make sure that your sole is planted firmly to the ground.
3. Drag your right knee to the side. You can either position the sole grounded on the floor, or lift the sole until only the blade rests on the surface.
4. Hold for five breaths before repeating the instructions with the opposite side.

MODIFICATIONS AND VARIATIONS

1. For a more advanced modification, you can lift your bend knee. Put your foot either on the inner thigh, knee, calf, or ankle. Try to place them on your ankles first, then gradually work your way up to your thighs if you can.
2. There are several options to adjust your hands based on your flexibility:
3. Stay relax on your lap.
4. On your waist.
5. Put together in front of the chest in praying pose.
6. Raised up to the ceiling.

INSTRUCTIONS

1. In the mountain pose, slightly shift your sitting to the side.

2. Start with the right side: bend your right knee backward without lifting your left leg. Point your right sole with active toes.

3. Grab either the instep or ankle of your right leg. Elevate it until your torso can stay upright and the nice stretch around your glutes and quadriceps are felt.

4. After holding for at least five breaths, come back to the mountain pose and start over with the left side.

COMMON MISTAKES TO AVOID

1. You have not actively engaged the muscle in your lower leg. This forces your hand to bear the weight disproportionally that can lead to an increase the risk of lateral torso bending. Maintain a straight upper body at all times.

GENERAL TIPS

1. When performing this pose, you can let your other hand (the one that isn't used to lift the lower leg) stay relaxed on your lap.

MODIFICATIONS AND VARIATIONS

1. If it feels too stiff to bend your knee deeply, wrap your instep with either a strap or towel. As long as your body remains elongated and there is no pain, it is acceptable only to lift your ankle slightly.

Scan the QR code or visit this URL to watch the video pose: https://balancedlivingbooks.com/chair-yoga-video-44

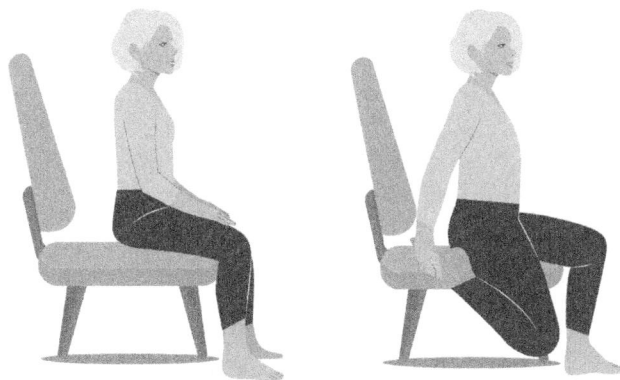

SCAN ME

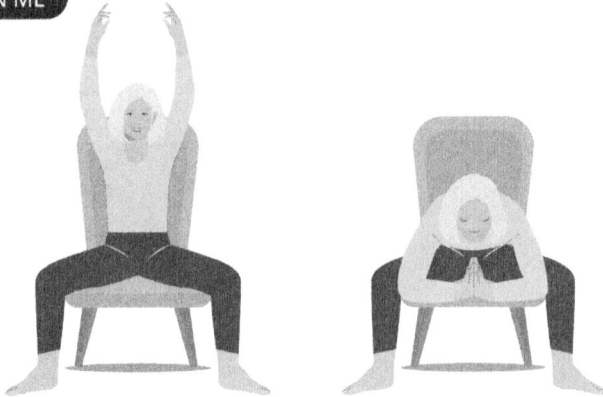

INSTRUCTIONS

1. Sit in the mountain pose.
2. Take one step to the right with your right foot and one step to the left with your left foot.
3. Take a deep beath and elongate your spine by raising your arms.
4. Exhale slowly and bend your torso forward.
5. Bring your hands together between your thighs. As you actively engage your arms, put a gentle pressure from your inner thighs toward your elbows. Maintain a neutral position for your head and neck.

COMMON MISTAKES TO AVOID

1. Spread your elbows sideways. Instead, attempt to give a slight pressure to your upper legs with your elbows.
2. Although our focus here is on the hip joints and upper leg muscles, it doesn't mean that we can loosen the spine's alignment. Keep it engaged to avoid curving. In addition, it's best not to rest your chest loosely on your lap or your seat. Aside from the risk of back curvature, it can make your arms feel heavier and unable to counterbalance the pressure from inner thighs.

MODIFICATIONS AND VARIATIONS

There are two adjustments you can make to this pose to lessen the strain or amp up the difficulty.

1. Stepping on yoga blocks is the recommended variation if your upper legs feel too stiff for doing the sequence above. Since elevating the footrest will reduce the stretch in the quadriceps, hip flexors, and hamstrings, you can focus on strengthening your inner thigh and arms muscles.
2. Putting your hands together in front of your chest isn't the only thing you can do to open your groin and hip joints. You can extend your right arm to your right side while simultaneously pressing your inner thigh. While doing this, raise your left arm to the ceiling in order to deepen the stretch for both groins. Remember to always do the same sequence for both sides.

INSTRUCTIONS

1. Step your feet out so they are farther than hip-width apart as you transition from the mountain pose.

2. Take a deep breath and elongate your spine.

3. While exhaling slowly, bring your torso forward until your chest is between your inner thighs.

4. Position your hands either nest to the inner edge of your feet or the middle front. Another more advance variation is to grab your ankle from behind and rest your palm on your shins.

Scan the QR code or visit this URL to watch the video pose: https://balancedlivingbooks.com/chair-yoga-video-46

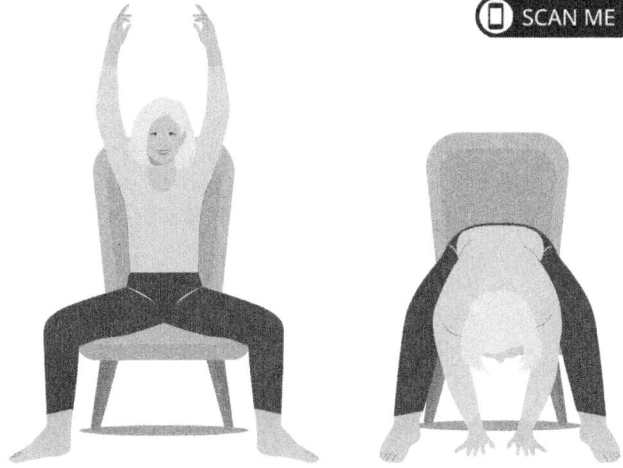

SCAN ME

Scan the QR code or visit this URL to watch the video pose: https://balancedlivingbooks.com/chair-yoga-video-47

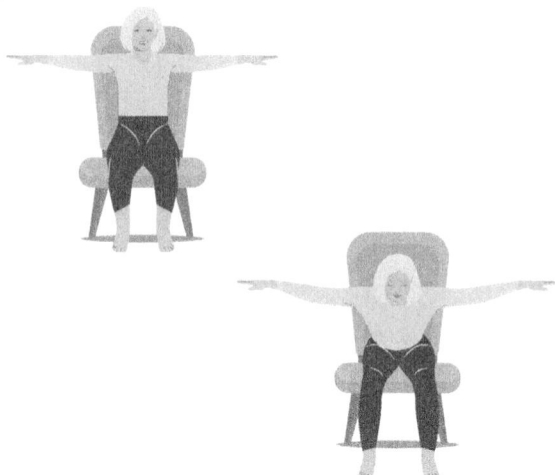

SCAN ME

INSTRUCTIONS

1. From the mountain pose, spread your arms sideways.

2. Bring your torso forward, parallel to the floor. However, don't rest your stomach or chest on your lap. Use your core to maintain the balance of your floating body.

3. Hold for a few seconds, then take some rest.

COMMON MISTAKES TO AVOID

1. Arms are not actively engaged. In order to reap the benefits from this pose, make sure that your arms are active.

2. Abs are not squeezed. Doing it will not only make it easy to maintain the balance but also to strengthen your core power.

3. When bending your torso, the spine isn't straightened. Keep elongating your back, so the weight isn't just concentrated in certain areas but is distributed evenly.

MODIFICATIONS AND VARIATIONS

1. Aside from bending your torso forward, you can add some side bending and twisting variations. Take that in separate sections to give your body a chance to recover in between modifications and catch some breath.

2. For example, after taking a break for a moment after bending your torso upward, you can go back to the mountain pose and spread your arms. Then, bend your waist laterally while maintaining your arms. If feasible, bend deeply until both your arms are almost making one straight line that is perpendicular to the ground. You can do the same steps for twisting as well.

3. Regardless of what variations you choose or how deep your body can go, make sure that your upper body isn't resting anywhere since this will undermine the objective to strengthening your core.

37. HALF LORD OF THE FISH POSE II (ARDHA MATSYENDRASANA II)

INSTRUCTIONS

1. From the mountain pose, extend your left leg forward and straighten the knee.

2. Flex your left foot and make sure the toes are actively engaged.

3. Bend your right knee and drag the ankle toward your left groin.

4. Inhale deeply and elongate your spine by raising your arms.

5. Exhale slowly and twist your torso to the left. Reach the outer sole of your left mid-foot with your right hand.

6. Stay there for five breaths. Release and repeat the steps for the opposite side.

Scan the QR code or visit this URL to watch the video pose: https://balancedlivingbooks.com/chair-yoga-video-48

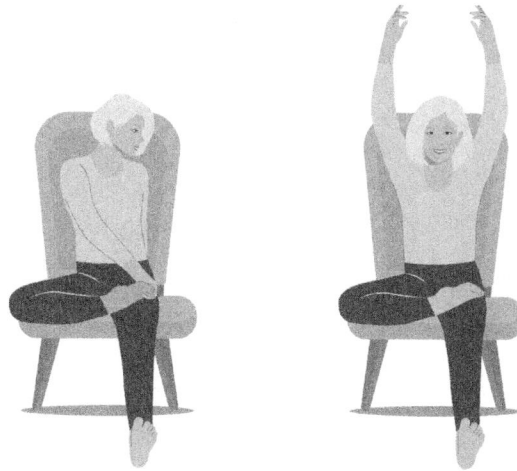

SCAN ME

COMMON MISTAKES TO AVOID

1. When bending your torso, hyperextend the knees. You can prevent this by using your core muscles to support your body weight. Doing so will reduce the tendency to press the ankle and put too much pressure on it—something that prone to locking the joints.

2. Not enough power to maintain the stability of the bent ankles. Always keep them actively engaged, so your ankles won't drop even if the pressure given by the hands isn't too forceful.

MODIFICATIONS AND VARIATIONS

1. You can use one or two straps if your hands are unable to reach both feet simultaneously.

2. If you are up for more challenge, you can do one additional step before releasing your outer sole. As your body is already in twisted state while still bending your right leg, you can grab the right ankle with your left hand from behind. In this state, you get the benefit of stretching the side of your torso, hips, hamstrings, and hip flexors simultaneously.

38. SEATED NOOSE POSE (PASASANA)

Scan the QR code or visit this URL to watch the video pose: https://balancedlivingbooks.com/chair-yoga-video-49

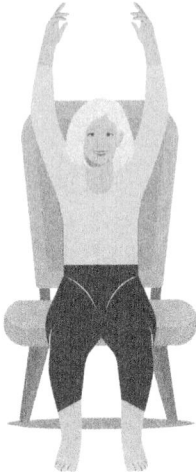

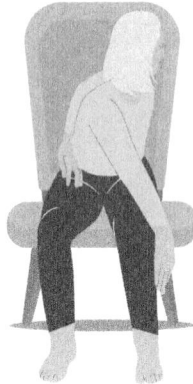

SCAN ME

INSTRUCTIONS

1. Sit in the mountain pose.

2. Raise your arms as you take a deep breath.

3. Lower down your right arm and bring it to the left side of your leg.

4. Drag your left arm to your right waist from the back. Alternatively, you can keep your left arm stretched upward.

5. Get a more intense twist by applying gentle pressure toward the outer side of your knee with your right elbow. You can do it until you feel your chest is more open.

GENERAL TIPS

1. If sitting right in the middle of the seat puts your knee joints against the front edge of the chair, slightly shift your bottom forward. When there is a gap between the back of your knee and the chair, it would be easier to position your hand next to your leg. Furthermore, it allows you to feel the deeper stretch coming from your elbow.

2. Gaze upward as you twist your torso.

VARIATION #1 – SITTING ON THE FLOOR WITH A CHAIR SUPPORTING YOUR LEGS

INSTRUCTIONS

1. Sit on a mat with a chair facing right in front of you. Set the distance not too far so that your hand can reach the backrest relatively easily.
2. Elevate your legs. Position your glutes in a way that enables your knees to straighten up.
3. Take a deep breath and elongate your spine. You can elevate your hands from sideways.
4. Exhale and slightly bend your torso toward the thighs.
5. Reach the backrest using both hands. Rest your head either on the shins or knees.
6. Stay there for five breaths before lowering your legs.

GENERAL TIPS

1. You can put a folded blanket to cushion your calves that pressing against the front edge of the chair.
2. If you are worried that somehow the chair will slip, use something heavy or line it with a rubber mat to hold the chair legs. Another alternative is to choose a location where you can lean the chair against a wall.

Scan the QR code or visit this URL to watch the video pose: https://balancedlivingbooks.com/chair-yoga-video-50

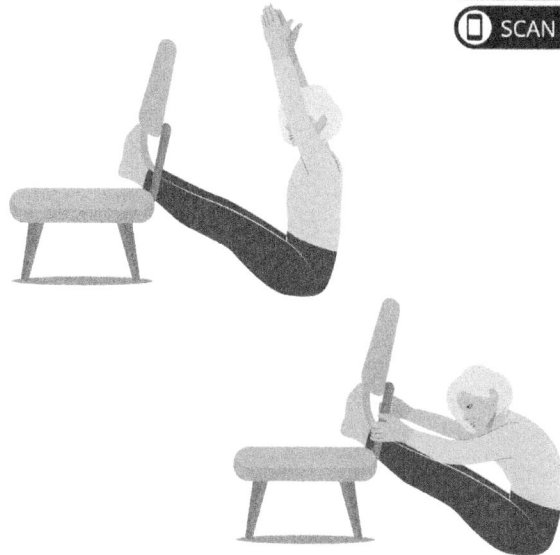

VARIATION #2: SITTING ON A CHAIR, CLOSE TO A WALL

INSTRUCTIONS

1. Set the chair away from the wall by about 20 inches (50 cm).
2. Sit in the mountain pose, facing the wall. Shift your sitting position closer to the backrest.
3. Raise your legs and lean them to the wall. To ease the process, you can lean your back against the backrest first, then grab your thighs with your hands. Make the necessary adjustments until your knees can be straightened upward.
4. Inhale deeply and raise your hands.
5. Exhale and draw your hands to reach your soles or ankles. Strengthen your grip by slightly bend your elbows. Rest your face on your shins.
6. Hold that position for at least five breaths. Feel the nice stretch on your back legs.

GENERAL TIPS

1. This action, which involves lifting your feet above your head, calls for a strong base and stability that is only recommended for advanced levels. For that reason, please practice with caution. If you are still having trouble elevating your legs or if your sitting isn't squared and stable enough, it would be best to avoid this pose.
2. The position of chair can be modified if you need something sturdy to support your calves. Instead of starting off from the usual mountain pose, you can turn the chair so that the backrest is facing the wall. Slowly and carefully, put your legs on top of the backrest. The back of your knees should rest steadily and your hands can easily grab the lower part of the backrest. Considering the nature of this variation, you may need someone to stand behind your back and give necessary support whenever you need it.
3. Since this variation requires a steadier foundation, it's recommended to try and get used to the first ones.

40. TORTOISE POSE (KURMASANA)

Scan the QR code or visit this URL to watch the video pose: https://balancedlivingbooks.com/chair-yoga-video-51

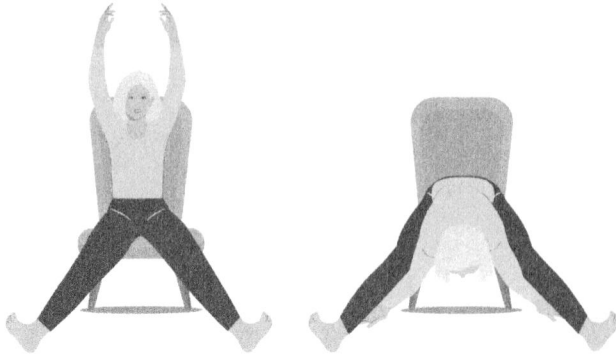

SCAN ME

INSTRUCTIONS

1. Sit in the mountain pose. Shift your sitting position slightly forward, closer to the front edge.
2. Open your legs wider than hip-width apart.
3. Take a deep breath and elongate your spine.
4. Exhale slowly and bend your torso forward until your hands can reach the floor.
5. Gradually drag your hands backward through the gap between your legs. You can place your hands either by grabbing the chair legs or slightly spread them to the outer side.

COMMON MISTAKES TO AVOID

1. Spread your knees sideways and loosen your legs' muscles.
2. Your forward bend shouldn't change the angle of your knees. Keep your legs in 90 degrees.

GENERAL TIPS

1. When bending, position your torso in between your thighs. Keep your legs' muscles actively engaged by gently press your waist.
2. Direct your gaze to between your hands, not backwards to keep the alignment between your spine, neck, and head.

RELAXATION AND MEDITATION

Savasana pose, or we can call it in English "the corpse pose", is the most common way for yogis to feel relaxed and connect with the higher power. As the name implies, savasana is done by lying still on a mat with closed eyes. We can modify that since we are focusing on using chairs.

1. Sit on a chair like the mountain pose. However, instead of positioning your hands on your lap, you can let them hang in a relaxed state on the sides of your body. Keep the palms facing forward without tensing any of your muscles.

2. If you finish your session in the bridge pose, you can do savasana in reclining position while elevating on a chair. Put your arms slightly further apart and be comfortable with your position.

3. You can use two chairs and do it in a forward bend position. Use some pillows to help your body at ease, so you don't have to stretch anywhere. Do it in a position where you feel relax the most: either by grabbing the pillow, resting your hands beneath your forehead, or hanging next to your torso.

GRATITUDE AND APPRECIATION

There are several ways we can do to incorporate gratitude and appreciation in our yoga practice:

1. Include reverence and thankfulness in your intention.

2. Use the time during breathing practice to have additional time for meditation. Normally, it would be easier to do because the hand movement and specific technique while breathing will help you be more focused on yourself, and obviously, preventing you from falling asleep or experiencing mind chatter.

3. Train yourself to be able to breathe deeper and longer. The more frequent you practice, the easier you feel to deepen the breathing rhythm.

4. Smile more often. This may look trivial and unnecessary, but smiling, even though the workout feel rigorous, will make your day lighter. It also encourage you to be able to be able to break down the negative thoughts that might block you from doing the movements that you can actually do.

5. Spend more time to do poses that focus on chest opening and stretching the throat. Both poses make it simpler to keep track of the rhythm of the breath because we will immediately pay attention to the movements of the chest and throat, which are the paths of the breath. Although actually, all yoga poses when performed correctly will help us become attentive of our breathing patterns.

In this enlightening chapter, we have dived into a wealth of valuable insights and practical guidance to help you go through chair yoga practice. Started by explanations on the importance of intentions, you have guided on how to craft meaningful weekly intentions, including some examples that you can implement directly or adjust here and there to make sure it is suitable for your circumstances.

Rolling on, this chapter also explores six essential breathing techniques, six invigorating warm-up practices to prepare your body for a productive yoga session, and a detailed breakdown of 40 poses that offer you a rich array of options to improve flexibility, strength, and balance, making it accessible for practitioners of all levels. This chapter concludes with some practical advice to relax, meditate, and cultivate gratitude for a holistic approach.

Ready to dive deeper into more practical routines? In the upcoming chapter, we will discover some recommendations for sequences and routines that are tailored based on your flexibility levels and specific goals, including weight loss and 10-minute practice. Turn the page and let's continue our journey through chair yoga!

CHAPTER 5
COMPLETE ROUTINES

Yoga begins right where I am—not where I was yesterday or where I long to be.
—Linda Sparrowe

In the previous chapter, we delved into dozens of breathing practices, warm-ups, and poses, along with various modifications that suit your abilities. While it is ideal to practice one complete set of yoga sessions that include all of those parts, you can also do them individually. However, exercise caution with more advanced poses that require warm-ups as a safety prerequisite.

For more practical consideration, you can also tailor your workout routine based on your objectives, for example, losing weight, exercising during your break, or improving flexibility. These are some ideas you can try. Most of them typically take around 20 minutes, although more focused ones usually require more time. If you want to exercise more than what is advised, you can either do some repetition or incorporate other poses that are mentioned in Chapter 4.

ROUTINES FOR BEGINNERS

Starting off exercise regimens with the beginners' sequence is the best option for those who have just begun their yoga journey or who have likely not practiced for a long time due to injuries, post-op recovery treatment, or other illnesses.

Total duration: 15–20 minutes

Optional props: a strap, a block, a pillow or a folded blanket.

Intentions: "To calm down my thoughts and manage mental chatter, I wish to slow down and be more flexible."

Be mindful with every discomfort you feel. It's okay to stop when you feel pain.

Scan the QR code or visit this URL to watch the video routine: https://balancedlivingbooks.com/cysr-01/

SCAN ME

Mountain Pose	3-Part Breathing	Head & Neck Stretching	Shoulders Stretching	Seated Butterfly with Yoga Block
15 sec	2 min / SCAN ME	30 sec x 2 Variations	30 sec	1 min

Wide-Legged Seated Forward Bend	Modified Chair Pose	Side Bending	Twisting
2 min	1 min	30 sec	30 sec x 2

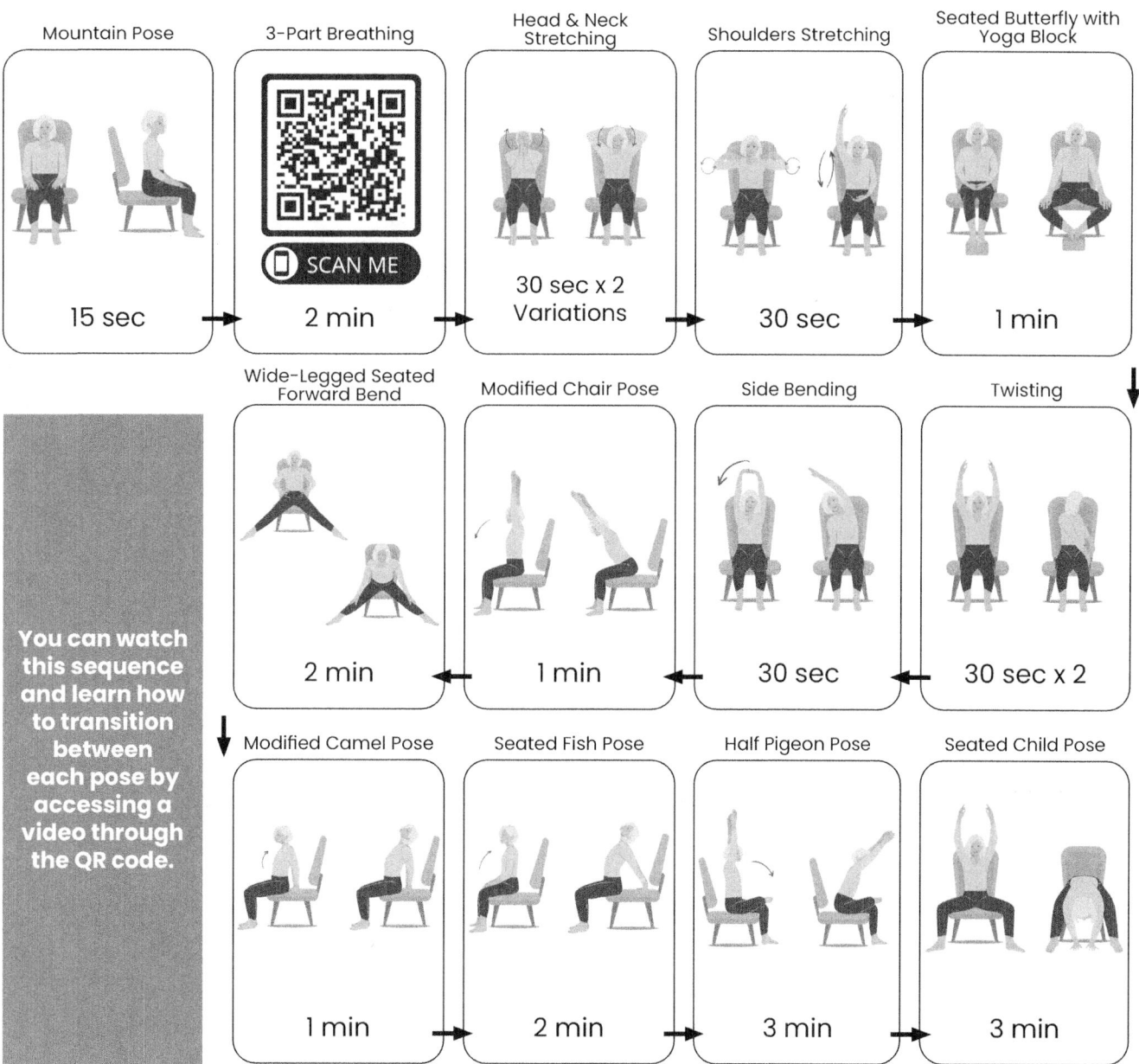

You can watch this sequence and learn how to transition between each pose by accessing a video through the QR code.

Modified Camel Pose	Seated Fish Pose	Half Pigeon Pose	Seated Child Pose
1 min	2 min	3 min	3 min

ROUTINES FOR INTERMEDIATE

Once you feel comfortable doing the beginner's routines without difficulties or panting breathing, you can increase the intensity by exercising at intermediate levels. You can combine both sequences as well, using the easier movements as a warm-up before performing the more difficult ones. At any time you feel this sequence is too challenging, you can always go back to the previous ones or substitute certain poses with others you deem more doable.

Total duration: 15-20 minutes

Optional props: two chairs, a strap, a pillow or a folded blanket.

Intention: "I want to explore the extent of my abilities and appreciate what I can do."

Reward yourself with a healthy meal and plenty of water.

Scan the QR code or visit this URL to watch the video routine:
https://balancedlivingbooks.com/cysr-02/

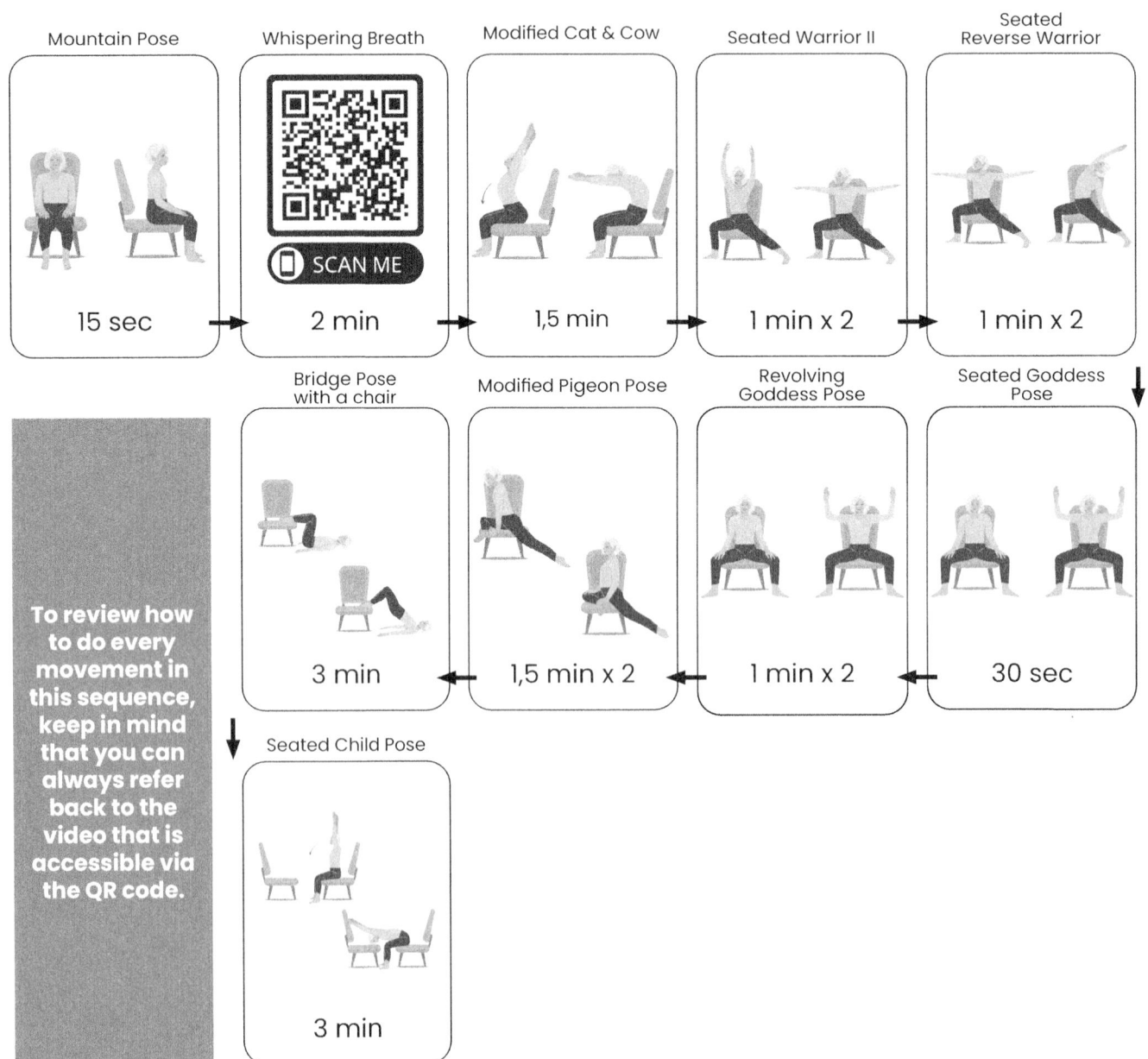

SCAN ME

Mountain Pose	Whispering Breath	Modified Cat & Cow	Seated Warrior II	Seated Reverse Warrior
15 sec	2 min (SCAN ME)	1,5 min	1 min x 2	1 min x 2

Bridge Pose with a chair	Modified Pigeon Pose	Revolving Goddess Pose	Seated Goddess Pose
3 min	1,5 min x 2	1 min x 2	30 sec

To review how to do every movement in this sequence, keep in mind that you can always refer back to the video that is accessible via the QR code.

Seated Child Pose

3 min

ROUTINES FOR LOSING WEIGHT

In general, routines for losing weight can be classified as intermediate, with more emphasis on movements that deeply engage core muscles. This emphasis is essential since having strong core muscles has a significant impact on your body's overall stamina, endurance, and stability. They can speed up the burning of visceral fat, particularly with ab-targeting activities.

Total duration: 20-25 minutes

Optional props: two chairs, a strap, a pillow or a folded blanket.

Intention: "Today, I'm going to pay greater attention to what my body tries to tell me."

Don't forget to smile and stay relaxed.

Scan the QR code or visit this URL to watch the video routine: https://balancedlivingbooks.com/cysr-03/

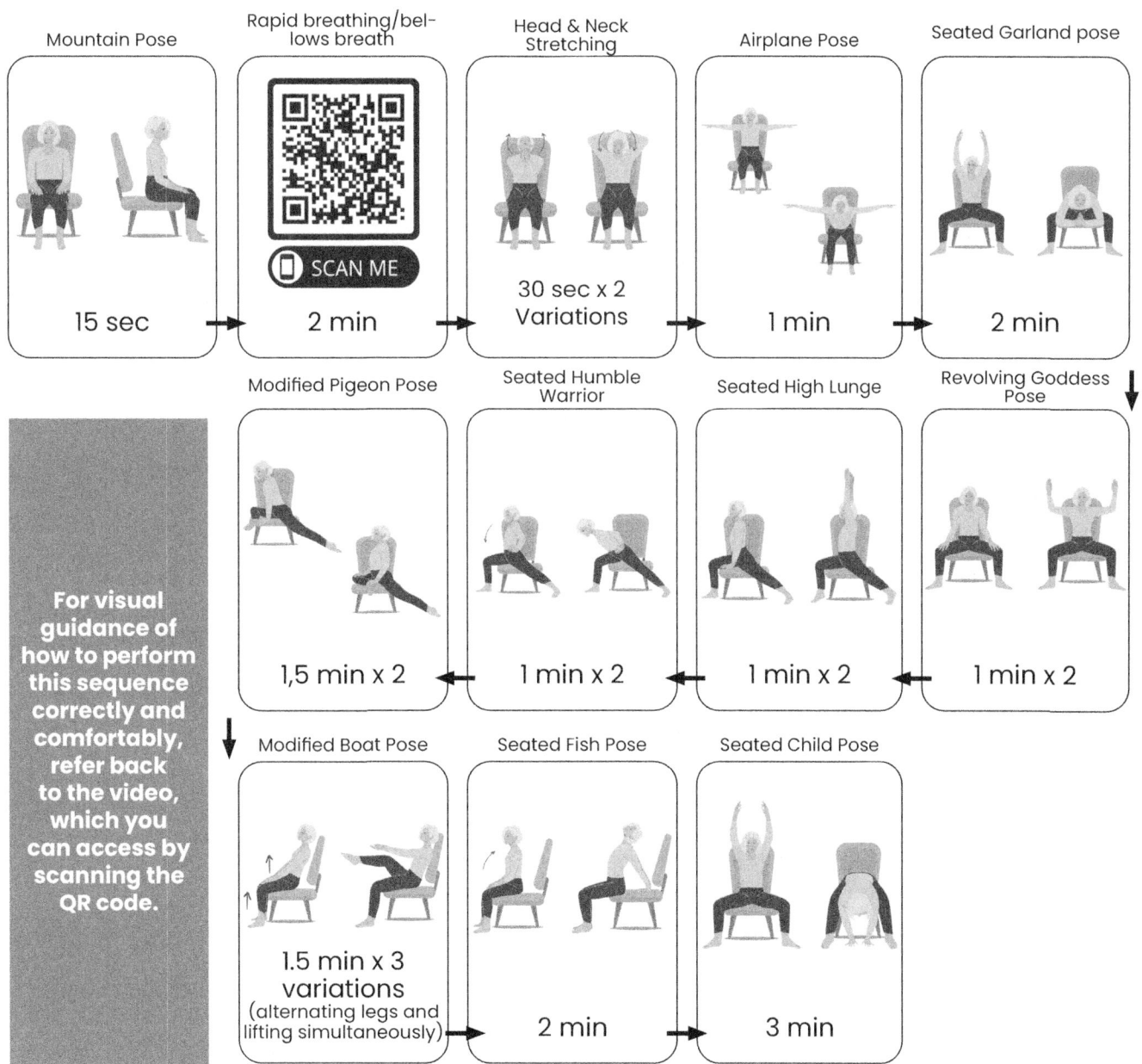

Mountain Pose	Rapid breathing/bellows breath	Head & Neck Stretching	Airplane Pose	Seated Garland pose
15 sec	2 min	30 sec x 2 Variations	1 min	2 min

	Modified Pigeon Pose	Seated Humble Warrior	Seated High Lunge	Revolving Goddess Pose
For visual guidance of how to perform this sequence correctly and comfortably, refer back to the video, which you can access by scanning the QR code.	1,5 min x 2	1 min x 2	1 min x 2	1 min x 2

Modified Boat Pose	Seated Fish Pose	Seated Child Pose
1.5 min x 3 variations (alternating legs and lifting simultaneously)	2 min	3 min

ROUTINES FOR 10-MINUTE YOGA SESSION

While most yoga sessions takes more than 30 minutes, it doesn't mean you can't make some modifications to finish them in no more than 10 minutes. Regardless of the quickness, it targets almost all vital muscles in yoga; so you will still get plenty of benefits. In addition, this sequence is suitable for everyone, including beginners and intermediate yogis. More advanced individuals who have more time can incorporate this into their sessions as warm-up sequences.

This 10-minute routine is perfect for giving your body a gentle workout in the morning, giving you an extra mood boost before doing your other daily activities. On the other hand, you can also do this before bed as a wrap-up for your day. Do it before you meditate, or write in your gratitude journal as a reminder to constantly be thankful for your physical well-being and to reflect on your accomplishments to date. Additionally, a brief workout can promote quicker and deeper sleep.

Total duration: 10 minute

Intention: "I wish to have more courage to take a small step that matters."

Even a small amount of time can be utilized for something joyful. Stretching your muscle is one of them.

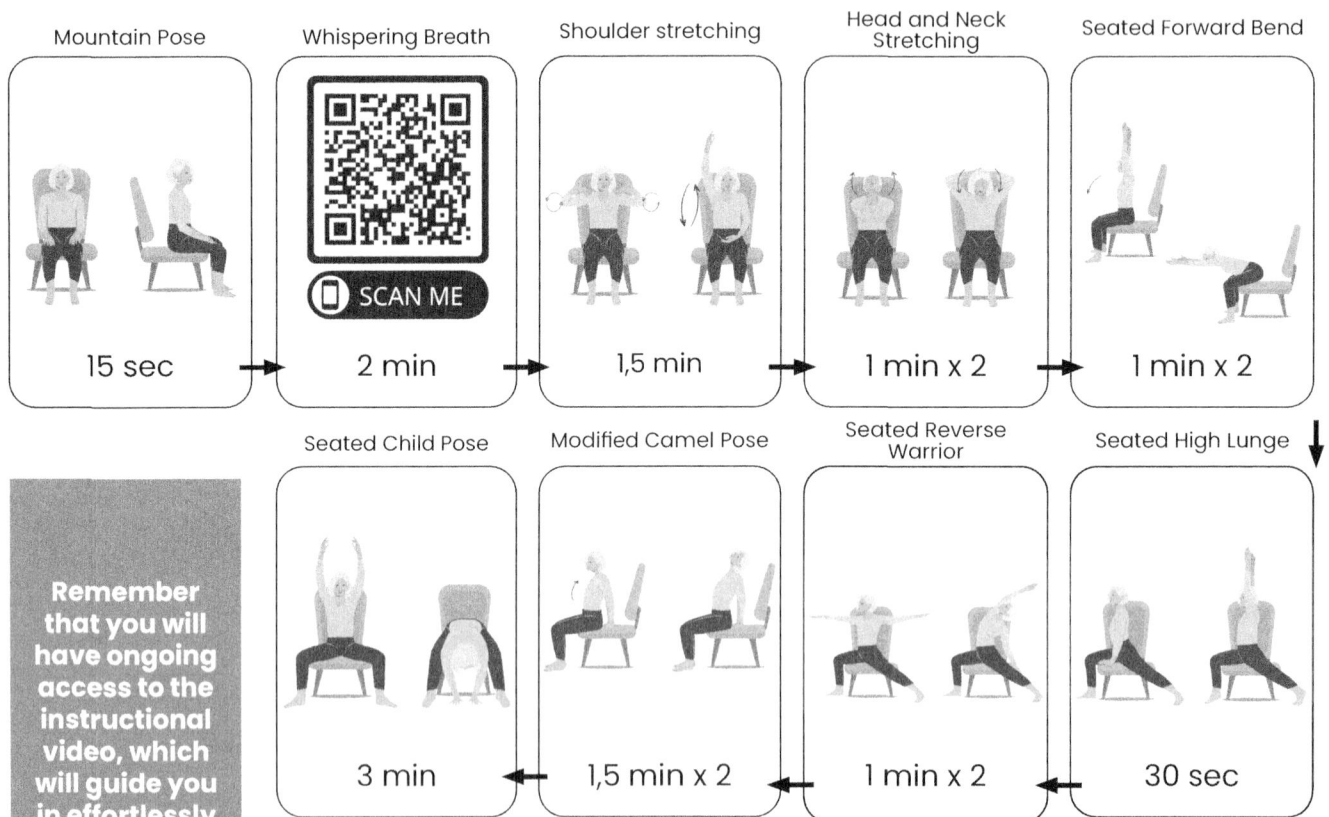

SCAN ME

Mountain Pose	Whispering Breath	Shoulder stretching	Head and Neck Stretching	Seated Forward Bend
15 sec	SCAN ME 2 min	1,5 min	1 min x 2	1 min x 2

Seated Child Pose	Modified Camel Pose	Seated Reverse Warrior	Seated High Lunge
3 min	1,5 min x 2	1 min x 2	30 sec

Remember that you will have ongoing access to the instructional video, which will guide you in effortlessly performing this sequence and transitioning between each pose seamlessly. You can scan the QR code.

Scan the QR code or visit this URL to watch the video routine: https://balancedlivingbooks.com/cysr-04/

CHAPTER 6:
THE 28-DAY CHALLENGE

Do the best you can, until you know better. Then, when you know better, do better.
—Maya Angelou

Up to this point, nearly all of the information you require to enhance your general wellness and lead a healthy lifestyle is currently within your grasp. Now, you have one additional tool to help you stay consistent in the long term and have gradual progression: the 28-day chair yoga challenge. This challenge will provide you with a better-controlled practice that will encourage you to practice yoga on a regular basis. Once you are able to reach the first milestone—let's say, the first seven days—you will be more challenged and driven to finish it till the very end. Moving forward, you will find it easier to see yoga as a part of your life.

With what you've learned thus far, this 28-day chair yoga challenge is designed to prevent muscle fatigue by varying postures on a daily basis. This means that, even though you exercise every day, your muscles will have proper time to heal because each day's workout menu targets a different set of body parts to train. However, although it's important to stay on track and be disciplined with the regimen, it's always best to listen to your body. Remember that the first principle of yoga is to practice with compassion and patience—make sure that your session doesn't feel hurtful. Don't stretch yourself too thin, and always take time to rest whenever your body needs it.

Beyond just doing the challenge, you can monitor your progress and reflect on your experience with a free Tracking Planner. We have crafted this planner to be your dedicated companion, so you can take your chair yoga practice to the next level. It's the perfect companion to enhance your 28-day challenge experience, as you will be able to take a proactive step towards achieving your wellness goals. You can download by scanning the QR code provided in the previous chapter.

By realizing how far you have accomplished, you will be able to easily remember your initial commitment and stay positive throughout the journey. To help you overcome excuses that may arise, you can pump up your spirit by celebrating small victories and being willing to embrace imperfection. You don't have to wait until the last day to appreciate your progress. Even on a daily basis, there is always something to be grateful for; whether it is the stretch that you are now able to do deeper, some new modifications that you are finally able to make, or something as simple as enjoying the sweat and getting good sleep afterwards. Bear in mind that it's your consistency that matters. Therefore, keep track of your progress and discover the life-changing potential of chair yoga!

HOW HABIT TRACKING CAN BE THE KEY TO MAKING A LASTING CHANGE

In our second chapter, we delved into the significance of feeling rewarded, and you can enhance this experience through the Tracking Planner you've acquired via the QR code at the beginning of the chapter. The benefits of using that planner go beyond simply marking your progress and providing a visual reminder of your commitment to your initial plan. It allows you to easily recognize and celebrate even the smallest of achievements that might otherwise go unnoticed without proper monitoring. This sense of accomplishment triggers the release of dopamine in your body, resulting in a heightened sense of happiness and boosted self-esteem as you conquer milestones you may never have thought possible. Since only dedicated individuals will undertake this challenge, you'll find yourself more motivated to maintain your consistent behavior, in this case, your chair yoga routine, in pursuit of another gratifying reward.

You can make that pleasant sensation stronger by rewarding yourself. Each week, celebrate a specific moment that you most enjoy. It can be spending a quality time with loved ones or taking a moment to breathe fresh air in nearby park—anything that help you recall "why" you chose to follow this path of life in the first place and appreciate the effort you've put in to get to where you are now with your routine workouts. In addition, you should celebrate even more after finishing this challenge since you have dedicated yourself to this journey, which is something that only truly committed people can achieve.

Now that we have embarked on a transformative 28-day challenge, you will see just how much room there is for personal development and overall well-being in just a month, only if you have the courage to push yourself. However, the journey to be a healthier individual doesn't end with the challenge itself. In the next chapter, you will find a comprehensive explanation about complete wellness that also addresses many important aspects in fostering a healthy lifestyle, such as mindful eating, nutritious diet, and other tips for mental health.

WEEK 1

DAY 1—CULTIVATING MINDFULNESS AND STABILITY

Intention: I want to be more courageous in facing my own thoughts, fears, and anxiousness.

Breathing practice: whispering breathing (2 min)

WARM-UPS:

1. Wrist stretching (4 variations x 30 secs = 2 minutes)
2. Ankle and toes stretching (3 minutes)
3. Lifting legs, but deeply engage your core muscle (2 minutes)

POSES:

1. Seated tree pose (1 minute)
2. Seated extended triangle pose (2 minutes)
3. Modified chair pose (1 minute)
4. Seated goddess pose (1 variation x 1 min = 1 minute)
5. Seated boat pose (3 minutes)
6. Seated child pose

TOTAL: 17–20 MINUTES

DAY 2—MORNING GLOW

Intention: I want to no longer be stuck in the past; I want to use the past as reflection to be able to move forward better.

Breathing practice: breathing with retention (3 min)

WARM-UPS:

1. Lifting legs (3 minutes)
2. Seated forward bend (2 variations x 1 min = 2 minutes)
3. Modified downward facing dog (2 minutes)

POSES:

1. Cat-and-cow (2 minutes)
2. Eagle pose (1.5 minutes)
3. Seated warrior I (3 minutes)
4. Reverse warrior (3 minutes)
5. Seated child pose

TOTAL: 20-25 MINUTES

DAY 3—TWIST AND UNWIND

Intention: I want to be more accepting of everything that happens in my life, regardless of whether it's something I planned or not.

Breathing practice: three-part breathing (1 minute)

WARM-UPS:

1. Twisting, with both hands grabbing the backrest (2 minutes)
2. Shoulders stretching (2 minutes)
3. Quadriceps and hamstrings stretching (2 minutes)

POSES:

1. Interlocked fingers and back bending (2 variations x 1.5 min = 3 minutes)
2. Seated forward bend with two chairs (2 minutes)
3. Sitting twist (3 minutes)
4. Revolved goddess pose (1 minute)
5. Relaxation and meditation

TOTAL: 15-19 MINUTES

DAY 4—RESTORATIVE YOGA

Intention: I want to calm the loud noise inside my head and take control over my overthinking.

Breathing practice: three-part breathing (2 minutes)

WARM-UPS:

1. Shoulders stretching (2 variations x 1 min = 2 minutes)
2. Head and neck stretching (3 variations x 1 min = 3 minutes)
3. Seated butterfly (1 minute)

POSES:

1. Hugging knees (2 minutes)
2. Garland pose (3 minutes)
3. Seated downward facing dog (1 minute)
4. Bridge pose (3 minutes)
5. Savasana with reclining back

TOTAL: 10-15 MINUTES

DAY 5—LIGHT HEAD SEQUENCE

Intention: I surrender; I want to release my attachment toward everything outside myself and be more grateful with what I have and what I can do.

Breathing practice: skull shining (2 minutes)

WARM-UPS:

1. Side bending with clasping hands (1 minute)
2. Wrist stretching (4 variations x 30 secs = 2 minutes)

POSES:

1. Half pigeon pose (2 minutes)
2. Modified camel pose (1 minute)
3. Seated fish pose (2 minutes)
4. Seated child pose

TOTAL: 10-12 MINUTES

DAY 6—ENERGIZING MORNING

Intention: I want to be free from feeling lethargic.

Breathing practice: rapid bellows breath (2 minutes)

WARM-UPS:

1. Head and neck stretching (2 variations x 1 min = 2 minutes)
2. Lifting legs with engaging core muscles (3 minutes)
3. Side bending (2 minutes)

POSES:

1. Wide-legged seated forward bend (2 variations x 1 min = 2 minutes)
2. Seated warrior II (2 minutes)
3. Seated humble warrior (2 minutes)
4. Seated extended side angle (2 minutes)
5. Airplane pose (3 minutes)
6. Boat pose (3 minutes)
7. Hero pose (2 minutes)
8. Relaxation and meditation

TOTAL 25-30 MINUTES

DAY 7—GENTLE CHEST OPENING

Intention: I want to be more flexible and have a big heart to accept what I can't change.

Breathing practice: alternate nostril breathing (3 minutes)

WARM-UPS:

1. Wrist stretching (2 variations x 1 min = 2 minutes)
2. Feet stretching (2 minutes)

POSES:

1. Modified cat-and-cow (2 minutes)
2. Interlocked fingers and back bending (2 variations x 1.5 min = 3 minutes)
3. Camel pose (2 minutes)
4. Seated eagle pose (2 variations x 1 min = 3 minutes)
5. Seated garland pose (2 minutes)
6. Bridge pose (2 minutes)
7. Savasana with reclining your back

TOTAL: 15-20 MINUTES

WEEK 2

DAY 8—CENTERING AND FIRMING UP FOUNDATION

Intention: I want to be present and mindful toward my alignment.

Breathing practice: skull shining (2 minutes)

WARM-UPS:

1. Shoulders stretching (1.5 minutes)

POSES:

1. High lunge (2 minutes)
2. Seated warrior II (2 minutes)
3. Chair pose (2 minutes)
4. Savasana on a chair

TOTAL: 10-12 MINUTES

DAY 9—ARMS AND ABS

Intention: I am stronger than I think.

Breathing practice: bellows breath (2 minutes)

WARM-UPS:

1. Modified downward facing dog (1 minute)
2. Side-bending with clasping hands (2 minutes)
3. Twisting with spread arms (2 minutes)

POSES:

1. Modified cat-and-cow with elongated arms (3 minutes)
2. Seated camel pose (2 minutes)
3. Modified goddess pose (3 variations x 1 min = 3 minutes)
4. Sitting twist (2 minutes)
5. Seated warrior I (2 minutes)
6. Seated reverse warrior (2 minutes)
7. Seated humble warrior (2 minutes)
8. Seated extended triangle pose (2 minutes)
9. Seated boat pose (3 minutes)
10. Half lord of the fish pose II (3 minutes)
11. Modified pigeon (2 minutes)
12. Tree pose (2 minutes)
13. Savasana on a chair

TOTAL: 40-45 MINUTES

DAY 10—STRESS RELIEF

Intention: I want to relieve stress by mending what has dragged me down.

Breathing practice: Take a regular deep breathing for five repetitions (2 minutes)

WARM-UPS:

1. Head and neck stretching (3 variations x 30 secs =1.5 minutes)
2. Wrist stretching (2 variations x 30 secs = 1 minute)
3. Ankle stretching (2 minutes)

POSES:

1. Seated butterfly (1 min)
2. Interlocked fingers and back bending (2 variations x 1 min = 2 minutes)
3. Seated fish pose (2 minutes)
4. Meditation and relaxation

TOTAL: 8-12 MINUTES

DAY 11—TWIST AND BIND

Intention: I want to release tension around the side of my torso.

Breathing practice: breathing with retention (2 minutes)

WARM-UPS:

1. Twisting with grabbing backrest (2 minutes)
2. Side bending (2 minutes)
3. Seated forward bend with two chairs (2 minutes)

POSES:

1. Noose pose (3 minutes)
2. Half lord of the fish pose II (3 minutes)
3. Revolved goddess pose (1.5 minutes)
4. Seated goddess poses involving core strength and side angle (4 minutes)
5. Sitting twist (3 minutes)
6. Garland pose (2 minutes)
7. Airplane pose with some side bending and twist variations (5 minutes)
8. Seated child pose and meditation

TOTAL: 30-35 MINUTES

DAY 12—FLEXIBILITY AND BALANCE

Intention: I want to be more confident with what I have.

Breathing practice: 3-part breathing (2 minutes)

WARM-UPS:

1. Lifting legs (2 minutes)
2. Ankle stretching (2 minutes)

POSES:

1. Seated tree pose (2 minutes)
2. Wide-legged forward bend (2 minutes)
3. Airplane pose (2 minutes)
4. Seated warrior II (2 minutes)
5. Interlocked fingers and back bending (2 minutes)

TOTAL: 15-20 MINUTES

DAY 13—OPENING HIPS

Intention: I want to be respectful and compassionate when my body is unable to do something.

Breathing practice: whispering breath (2 minutes)

WARM-UPS:

1. Seated butterfly (1 minute)
2. Lifting legs (2 minutes)
3. Quadriceps and hamstring stretching (3 minutes)

POSES:

1. Seated forward bend with two chairs (2 minutes)
2. High lunge (2 minutes)
3. Half pigeon pose (2 minutes)
4. Modified pigeon pose (2 minutes)
5. Seated garland pose (2 minutes)
6. Seated child pose

TOTAL: 18-20 MINUTES

DAY 14—UPPER BODY STRENGTH

Intention: I want to train my endurance with compassion.

Breathing practice: whispering breath (2 minutes)

WARM-UPS:

1. Shoulders stretching (3 minutes)
2. Hugging knees (2 minutes)
3. Interlocked fingers and back bending, with namaste on the back (4 minutes)

POSES:

1. Seated eagle pose (2 minutes)
2. Seated warrior I (2 minutes)
3. Seated reverse warrior (2 minutes)
4. Seated triangle pose (2 minutes)
5. Seated chair pose (2 minutes)

TOTAL: 20-25 MINUTES

WEEK 3

DAY 15—STRENGTHENING THIGHS AND GLUTES

Intention: Balance is something I'm working on, both on and off the chair.

Breathing practice: bellows breath (2 minutes)

WARM-UPS:

1. Ankles and toes stretching (2 minutes)
2. Lifting knees (2 minutes)
3. Hugging knees (2 minutes)

POSES:

1. Cat-and-cow with extended arms (2 minutes)
2. Seated camel pose (2 minutes)
3. Seated happy baby pose (3 minutes)
4. Tortoise pose (2 minutes)
5. Seated noose pose (2 minutes)
6. Intense forward bend (4 minutes)

TOTAL: 20-25 MINUTES

Intention: I want to let go of the past and embrace the unknown of tomorrow.

Breathing practice: alternate nasal breathing

WARM-UPS:

1. Seated cat and cow (2 minutes)
2. Interlocked fingers and back bending with namaste on the back (3 minutes)
3. Side bending (3 minutes)

POSES:

1. Twisting (2 pose)
2. Seated camel pose (2 minutes)
3. Modified boat pose (2 minutes)
4. Seated reverse warrior (2 minutes)
5. Seated humble warriors (2 minutes)
6. Fish pose (2 minutes)
7. Bridge pose (2 pose)

TOTAL: 20-25 MINUTES

DAY 17—LOWER LIMBS STRENGTH

Intention: Make my foundation steadier.

WARM-UPS:

1. Feet and ankle stretching (4 minutes)
2. Lifting legs (2 minutes)
3. Hugging knees (2 minutes)
4. Quadriceps and hamstring stretching (3 minutes)

POSES:

1. Modified downward facing dog (1 minute)
2. Seated forward bend with chairs (3 minutes)
3. Seated warrior II (2 minutes)
4. Modified extended side angle (2 minutes)
5. Half pigeon pose (2 minutes)
6. Savasana

TOTAL: 25-30 MINUTES

DAY 18—MODIFIED SUN SALUTATION

Intention: Take some rest, hydrate, and enjoy every movement.

POSES:

1. Seated child pose (1 minute)
2. Seated camel pose (2 minutes)
3. Seated forward bend (2 minutes)
4. Seated garland pose (2 minutes)
5. Modified downward facing dog (2 minutes)
6. Relaxation and meditation

TOTAL: 8-10 MINUTES

Intention: Realizing that sometimes my mind is the one that limits my mobility, but wisely acknowledging that I need limits to ensure safety.

WARM-UPS:

1. Seated downward facing dog (1 minute)
2. Cat-and-cow with extended arms (3 minutes)

POSES:

1. Seated forward bend with variation (3 minutes)
2. Seated high lunge (2 minutes)
3. Seated warrior II (2 minutes)
4. Seated goddess pose with side bending and core strength (4 minutes)
5. Modified extended triangle pose (2 minutes)
6. Modified pigeon pose (2 minutes)
7. Seated garland pose with extending your arms (4 minutes)
8. Seated happy baby pose (2 minutes)
9. Seated child pose

TOTAL 25-30 MINUTES

DAY 20—WIND-RELIEVING SEQUENCE

Intention: Stay energized and positive to every living being around me.

WARM-UPS:

1. Shoulders stretching (3 minutes)
2. Head and neck stretching (3 minutes)

POSES:

1. Modified downward facing dog (1 minute)
2. Modified extended triangle pose (2 minutes)
3. Reverse warrior (2 minutes)
4. Seated forward bend with two chairs (3 minutes)

TOTAL: 10-15 MINUTES

DAY 21—RISE AND SHINE

Intention: Listen to my body and be respectful to what my body needs.

WARM-UPS:

1. Wrist stretching (3 minutes)
2. Quadriceps and hamstrings stretch (2 minutes)
3. Lifted legs (2 minutes)

POSES:

1. Seated warrior II (2 minutes)
2. Wide-legged forward bend (2 minutes)
3. Goddess pose and 3 other variations (5 minutes)
4. Reverse warrior (2 minutes)
5. Bridge pose (3 minutes)
6. Savasana with reclining back

TOTAL 20-25 MINUTES

WEEK 4

DAY 22—DETOX AND CLEANSE

Intention: I want to cleanse my body and thoughts from negativity; so there will be room for more positivity.

WARM-UPS:
1. Twisting (2 minutes)
2. Side bending (2 minutes)

POSES:
1. Seated goddess pose with side bending and core strength variations (5 minutes)
2. Revolved goddess pose (3 minutes)
3. Pigeon pose (2 minutes)
4. Sitting twist (2 minutes)
5. Airplane pose with basic and twisting variation (4 minutes)
6. Seated forward bend (1 minute)
7. Seated child pose

TOTAL: 20-25 MINUTES

DAY 23—EVENING RELAXATION

Intention: I want to have a restful night, so I can wake up feeling more energized the morning after.

Breathing practice: three-part breathing (2 minutes)

POSES
1. Seated forward bend (1 minute)
2. Seated butterfly pose, with a pillow or blanket as a substitute for yoga block (1 minute)
3. Half pigeon (3 minutes)
4. Sitting twist (3 minutes)
5. Interlocked fingers with back bending (2 minutes)

TOTAL: 10 MINUTES

DAY 24—FLEXIBILITY THROUGH SIDE BENDING

Intention: I embrace joy and adapt gracefully to life's changes.

WARM-UPS:
1. Shoulders stretching (4 minutes)
2. Side bending with clasping fingers (3 minutes)
3. Ankle and feet stretching (4 minutes)

POSES:
1. Seated eagle pose (2 minutes)
2. Modified chair pose (2 minutes)
3. Modified extended triangle pose with hands extended to the ceiling (3 minutes)
4. Seated garland pose (3 minutes)
5. Seated child pose

TOTAL: 20-25 MINUTES

DAY 25—ELEVATE AND UPLIFT

Intention: My former self is the only person I wish to use as a benchmark.

Breathing practice: bellows breath

WARM-UPS:

1. Lifted legs (2 minutes)
2. Feet and ankle stretching (3 minutes)
3. Seated butterfly (1 minute)
4. Wrist and shoulders stretching (3 minutes)

POSES:

1. Quadriceps and hamstrings stretching, followed by bending and straightening legs without lowering them (4 minutes)
2. Hugging knees (2 minutes)
3. Sitting twist (3 minutes)
4. Seated forward bend with two chairs (3 minutes)
5. Half pigeon pose (2 minutes)
6. Modified pigeon pose (3 minutes)
7. Modified boat pose (3 minutes)
8. Bridge pose (3 minutes)
9. Savasana in a reclined back

TOTAL: 30-35 MINUTES

DAY 26—EMBRACING SELF-LOVE AND SELF-ACCEPTANCE

Intention: I will always endeavor not to let external chaos interfere with my inner vitality.

Breathing practice: combining alternate nasal breathing (2 minutes) followed by whispering breath (2 minutes)

WARM-UPS:

1. Head and neck stretches (2 minutes)
2. Wrists stretching (2 minutes)
3. Feet and ankles stretching (2 minutes)

POSES:

1. Seated wide-legged forward fold (2 minutes)
2. Half pigeon pose (2 minutes)
3. Tree pose (1 minute)

TOTAL: 10-15 MINUTES

DAY 27—RECHARGE ENERGY WITH WARRIOR POSES

Intention: I want to replenish my vitality to be more positive about living my best life.

Breathing practice: starting from three-part breathing for three to four cycles, then continuing to bellow breath (3 minutes)

WARM-UPS:

1. Ankle and toes stretching (3 minutes)
2. Lifting legs (2 minutes)
3. Hugging knees (2 minutes)
4. Sitting twist (2 minutes)

POSES:

1. Modified extended triangle pose (2 minutes)
2. Seated high lunge (2 minutes)
3. Seated reverse warrior (2 minutes)
4. Seated humble warrior (2 minutes)
5. Back to reverse warrior (2 minutes)
6. Modified extended side angle (2 minutes)
7. Half lord and fish pose II (2 minutes)
8. Half pigeon pose (2 minutes)
9. Seated forward pose (1 minute)
10. Savasana in a seated position

TOTAL: 30-35 MINUTES

Intention: I calm my mind with every breath I inhale and expel negativity with every breath I exhale.

Breathing practice: combining three-part breathing (3 minutes) and bellows breath (2 minutes)

1. Warm-ups:
2. Shoulders stretching, with practicing whispering breath (2 minutes)
3. Seated eagle pose (2 minutes)

POSES:

1. Seated cat-and-cow with extended elbows (2 minutes)
2. Hero pose (3 minutes)
3. Happy baby pose (2 minutes)
4. Seated fish pose (2 minutes)
5. Bridge pose (2 minutes)
6. Relaxation and meditation

TOTAL: 15–20 MINUTES

CHAPTER 7:
COMPLETE WELLNESS

If you set your goals ridiculously high and it's a failure, you will fail above everyone else's success.
— James Cameron

Just like any other physical activity, it takes supporting efforts to ensure that your yoga practice actually has the positive impact on your body and mind that you expect. Mindful and healthy eating play a crucial role in understanding the connection between yoga and diet, and to what extent both of them contribute to the achievement of complete wellness.

HOW YOUR YOGA PRACTICE IS CORRELATED TO HEALTHY EATING

If previously we discussed that yoga is an ideal go-to option for those who want to be healthier, it's also proven that practicing yoga can encourage people to be mindful of their daily life choices, including the tendency to eat healthily, in contrast to those who never engage in yoga and have a poor diet.

When your body is habituated to exercise, you put emphasis on the awareness of breathing patterns, which will unconsciously lead you to better regulate your attachment and emotion to eating. You will notice that now you can control your impulse to crave something sweet or binge-eating—regardless of whether you have a plan to lose weight.

WHAT IS MINDFUL EATING AND WHY IT IS IMPORTANT

In general, mindful eating is a branch of mindfulness—the state when you are fully aware of your feelings and thoughts and any occurrence surrounds you—that is related to eating. Therefore, this practice encourages people to enjoy the meal from every aspect, from the appearance, the taste, the smell, and everything else that you can observe through your senses. In addition to having a good effect on how you feel food, exploring every physical, sensory, and emotional component of any food you are going to eat can also help you cultivate a sense of gratitude for it. Since we already learned about the importance of practicing gratitude and appreciation on a daily basis, a simple act of eating with full attention can help you achieve that.

When there are no outside distractions at mealtimes, people are more likely to make healthy food choices rather than consuming food haphazardly for the sake of eating. Additionally, by indulging your senses, you will train your taste receptors to recognize and enjoy the natural sweetness and other flavors of less processed foods, which may become considerably less noticeable when the item is overheated or combined with additional ingredients. As a result of your heightened food sense, you will feel full more quickly and opt for a smaller serving size instead of sneaking through a whole bag of chips during a binge-watch. Over time, these dietary behavioral adjustments will lead to a more stable body weight and an increased level of energy for physical activity, including practicing exercise.

By practicing mindful eating, you will be able to attain four awareness goals: what you are eating, how you are going to consume it, how much you can eat without going overboard, and why you chose to eat it. These goals not only allow you to experience the taste in a manner that you cannot when you choose to divert your attention from your meal, but they also help you develop self-control by suppressing your negative, impulsive behavior related to food. For instance, you can stop eating right when you've satisfied yourself because your body is able to detect the signal when you feel full more efficiently. On the other side, since you won't take food more than you can consume, this behavior can help prevent food waste. The same applies to knowing why you are eating that particular item. This takes into account not only the nutrition but also the environmental effects. You are probably going to be more aware of which foods have less of an impact on the environment as you are driven to choose healthful foods rather than highly processed foods that have lost nutrients.

With this concept, unfortunately some people tend to misinterpret mindful eating as being strict to yourself in terms of calories intake that lead to perception that mindful eating prevent people from the pleasurable and social aspects of eating; for example, by enjoying the good companies of others. So, what are the boundaries that determine whether people eat mindfully or not?

The antithesis of mindful eating, mindless eating, occurs when a person eats too quickly to the point that their brain fails to comprehend the hunger and fullness signals coming from their digestive organs, is too preoccupied to enjoy their food, or is unable to set aside time to eat without being glued to their phone screens. In this sense, those who eat for purposes other than hunger, such as when they eat to make up for emotional distress or other strong emotions, can be classified as mindless eating as well. When weighed against all the advantages of mindful eating, mindless eating will not allow us to attain that. In this way, dining with friends doesn't have to be considered thoughtless since it can actually improve the experience of the meal you're eating. On the other hand, mindless eating occurs when you use your phone to text or talk since it takes your focus away from your food. This distinction arises as a result of the direct connection between social eating and the development of a sense of appreciation for life and interpersonal connections, as well as the maintenance of emotional support and the mitigation of the effects of loneliness. For this reason, even though the food and atmosphere aren't particularly fancy, there's a greater likelihood that you will appreciate it more when you're with other people.

NUTRITION, VITAMINS, AND THE IMPORTANCE OF HEALTHY FOODS

Good nutrition is one of the most basic pre-requisites for your body to have energy for doing activities, maintaining focus, and preventing diseases from attacking your immune system.

There are two types of nutrition that our bodies need to be able to stay healthy: macro and micronutrient. The energy that supplies our muscles, tissues, and internal organs come from carbohydrates, fat, and protein—all are belong to macronutrient category. On the other hand, we also need vitamins and minerals that are categorized as micronutrients, although the amount may be much fewer compared to the needs for macronutrients. Due to this amount difference, people who eat less mindfully may have higher chance to have nutrition imbalance because they may less concern with the content of what they eat.

Although nutritional imbalances are detrimental for all people, they are especially severe for seniors over 50. Since the building blocks of muscles, nerves, tissues, and brains are found in diet, therefore deficits will have a major impact on your capacity to perform daily tasks, let alone comfortably complete an exercise routine.

Compared to younger people, often have slower metabolisms and other physiological changes that make them more vulnerable to health problems. According to research (Evans, 2005), American people over 65 years old were at more risk for undernutrition due to only consuming fewer than 1000 calories per day. Studies have shown that Americans over 65 who consume less than 1000 calories per day are more likely to suffer from undernutrition.

Unfortunately, as many of them also experience inadequate nutrient absorption, simply increasing the intake cannot always be the solution. Moreover, the more we age, the less we need calories since the needs to maintain muscle mass won't be as much as younger people in their productive age due to reduced activities. However, be careful if this condition leads to other problems, including sudden weight changes, loss of appetite, extreme fatigue, and other unexplained pain or bodily discomfort, as medical intervention may be needed immediately.

If being left unaddressed, this issue can affect vision health, bone density, cognitive and physical conditions, as well as lower immune system. Because these nutrients are crucial for seniors but frequently unfulfilled, think about including some of these items either daily or as frequently as feasible to avoid the worst-case scenario:

- Fatty fish like salmon, mackerel, and anchovies to fulfil the needs of omega 3 and animal proteins.
- Fibers and antioxidants from berries and other vibrant colors–fruit.
- Food high in B12, including sardines, clams, beef, tuna, eggs, and fortified dairy products.

- Leafy vegetables for plant-based proteins, vitamin A and C, calcium, and other essential minerals that reduce the risk of inflammation.
- Cruciferous vegetables like cauliflower, broccoli, Brussel sprout, and radishes. This food is essential due to high content of vitamins, phytochemicals, and fibers.
- Dairy products like cheese, yogurts, dairy and plant-based milk to get enough calcium and vitamin D.
- Whole grains for B-complex vitamins, insoluble fibers, and minerals to control cholesterol levels.

TIPS FOR A BALANCED AND NUTRITIOUS DIET

While there are lots of recommendations and advice on how to ensure a balanced nutrient intake, there is no one-size-fit-all approach that can't answer everyone's bodies. However, unless there is certain specific conditions that need more medical attention, there are some general guidelines for nutritious diets that are applicable to everyone:

1. Eat a wide range of food every day.

Attempt to have a balanced proportion of every type of food, including vegetables, fruits, beans and legumes, wholegrain, fish, meat, milk, and so on. The different nutrients in each type of food can help your body fulfill its nutritional needs.

2. Limit sugar, salt, fat, oil, and preservatives intake.

While all the options out there seem impossible for people to get free from those additives, it doesn't mean we can't do anything to limit the negative impact. If you buy packaged food, always check the ingredients and choose the ones with fewer additives per serving.

3. Drink adequate water.

Attempt to drink tap or mineral water rather than flavored ones whenever possible. This can be the cheapest and easiest way to keep our body fresh while also preventing any excess calories.

4. Take supplements if needed.

To compensate for the lack of certain specific nutrients, you may consider taking supplements. However, proceed with cautions since too many supplements may have another negative impact as well. Consult with your physicians or take a blood test first to make sure what kind of supplement you need.

FOSTERING HABITS TO MAINTAIN MENTAL HEALTH

As mentioned in Chapter 2, we have discussed that practicing self-care is important if you want to incorporate new healthy habit in your life. In this sense, there is a direct correlation between the success of fostering habits and your current state of mental health. You can do some tips below to help you maintaining and preparing your psychological state to be ready to adhere with the new goals your intent to achieve.

1. Adequate sleep

There is mounting data that suggests individuals who get enough good-quality sleep also tend to be happier and more productive, despite the opinions of some experts who maintain that the relationship between sleep and mental health is complicated. On the other hand, people who have issues with their mental health are most likely suffering from sleep deprivation as well, regardless of whether or not both of them have direct causality.

2. Purposeful walks

Walking isn't just beneficial for your health—it does magic for your mental health as well. Psychologically speaking, it affects positively to sleeping pattern, stress regulation, alertness, and mood. The other impact that are most obvious are the ones that related to physical, such as increased energy, improved stamina, and less fatigue.

Our hearts become more adept at pumping blood quickly when we walk. Faster blood pumping also results in enhanced blood flow, which improves the efficiency of oxygen and nutrition delivery to all vital organs. This isn't just refreshing and invigorating; it also elevates your mood since improved oxygen flows help your central nervous system—the nerves responsible for fight-and-flight response—to be calmer.

3. Positive connections with others

Having a close social circle has a bunch of benefits. The social support they provide, especially when you may feel alone, has a strong connection with reduced depression, less isolation, and more brain activation, leading to better memory and cognitive skills.

4. Continuous learning

Apparently, "lifelong learner" isn't just a saying to sharpen cognitive skills but also to improve your mental health as well. When we continuously challenge ourselves to learn something new, it will give us a new sense of purpose while also fostering self-confidence simultaneously. It's not about how adept you are in your new fields, but more about how you handle the challenge you are facing and the pleasant feeling every time you can accomplish something, no matter how small it is. This sense of accomplishment gives you the same feeling as we have discussed earlier in relation to the dopamine flush when you achieve something, and this leads you to be more determined to stick with the pattern. Combining both of them will improve your chance of fostering a workout routine as you become more familiar with putting goals and plans on your mind.

Throughout this chapter, we have delved into the profound connection between incorporating yoga routines into your daily life and the interplay of nurturing mental health and self-care. By emphasizing the nature of overall wellness, we have shed light on how a balanced approach to both physical and psychological aspects can lead us to a better lifestyle that we have planned to accomplish. Turn the page and embark on this book's conclusion; we will tie together all the tips and advice we have explored from the first chapter.

CONCLUSION

Like any other life-changing new routine, practicing chair yoga is a long—sometimes arduous—journey, yet the physical and mental transformation you will benefit along the process makes all the efforts pay off. In times when you feel tired and lose sight of what you are trying to achieve, reflect again on the intention-making practice and refresh your memory about what made you choose this path in the first place. Once you realize that this is one of the ideal gateways to improved mobility, regulating emotional issues, regaining independence, and a deeper connection to your inner thoughts, you will also realize how rich and precious it is to improve overall well-being.

Throughout every chapter in this book, you have delved into a wide range of movements, how to breathe mindfully, and tips to stay committed to practicing chair yoga. All tips, guidance, and challenges spread across seven chapters are designed to prepare your stepping stones to a healthier, more harmonious you. Therefore, the content is balanced between practical step-by-step instructions and science-backed explanations that provide a valid foundation for what and why you need to do all those things. In the end, this effort reflects your dedication to enhancing your health and quality of life, as well as your persistence and resilience to become more independent regardless of your starting point. Hopefully, this book depicts a clearer path toward your life-changing transformation.

Let's take a look and highlight the key takeaways we have delved into about chair yoga, the formation of healthy habits, and how both of them contribute to an improved quality of life.

1. Be aware and compassionate with your body but stay open to opportunities to challenge your body to do new things.

People's responses can vary when they confront the limitations of their own bodies. Some individuals might refrain from attempting anything at all, while others might exhibit greater resilience, attempting to push their boundaries before reaching their ultimate limits. These diverse reactions are entirely reasonable, shaped by our past experiences, self-perception, compassionate levels to our own bodies, as well as our current mental state.

It's crucial to recognize that regardless how limited your mobility is, it doesn't mean that it should dim your light for pursuing any means for healing and recovery, including trying a new workout routine. At the end of the day, there remains ample opportunity to explore and break through the barriers that may have previously deterred you from trying something new without disregarding any health and safety precautions based on your individual's circumstances.

A lot of variations and modifications in this book are crafted based on this realization. You may think you can't do a certain pose just because that's not what people with stiff body do. Embrace the opportunity to try something new, and soon you will be amazed to how far actually your body can go through.

2. Be accountable to yourself.

Setting up intentions and preparing a safe environment to practice chair yoga is one thing, but being accountable to yourself and staying committed to your plan is the other. Find a way that suits your style best, so you can keep incorporating this healthy routine until you are able to do that automatically.

3. Your mental state is as important as your physical body.

When attempting to establish healthy habits until they become second nature, people often become trapped in the belief that the first thing that needs to be trained and changed to relinquish its sedentary behaviors is our physical body. While it is true that moving your body and maintaining a nutritious diet are essential for maintaining stamina and flexibility, a significant lifestyle transformation also needs to be balanced with paying more attention to your mental health, spiritual needs, and emotional support from your surroundings. This is where self-care and overall wellness come into play in the process of habit formation and cultivating a healthier body; they act as the nurturing foundation upon which lasting change can thrive.

4. Listen to your body and be compassionate.

It's crucial to understand that our minds frequently place restrictions on what the body may perform. Perceptions, views, and ways of thinking play a major role in influencing our decisions in life in a variety of situations. For example, it can influence whether you choose to live a comfortable, sedentary life with long-term risks or a healthier, more physically demanding lifestyle that feels rewarding.

However, it is even more important to listen to the signals your body sends you when you do something new. How your body reacts to exercising at a higher intensity than usual, such as excessive fatigue, dizziness, shaking, or nausea, is your body's way of telling you to stop and rest. Being compassionate to what your body needs isn't a form of selfishness and laziness; it's a proof that you respect and considerate what's best for your body.

5. Just get started!

Now that you already have all the information to get started, it's time to practice. If planning for a full session seems daunting, you can start with the 10-minute routine mentioned in Chapter 5. Give yourself a few minutes to try and monitor what you feel. Your body will thank you later for the invigorating sensation of loosening the stiff muscles, and as long as you keep practicing, you will arrive at the transformation you once felt far away.

When you encounter moments of demotivation while maintaining your routines, remember that you have the videos accessible via the QR codes placed throughout this book to offer you valuable support. Serving as your ideal companions, these videos have been thoughtfully crafted to guide you through every routine while also helping you feel less alone on this journey.

Thank you for joining me on this transformative journey. It's been my privilege to walk you through improving your wellness. I hope that my personal and professional background, accumulated over a decade of helping people discover the best version of themselves through yoga, can assist you in regaining flexibility, strength, relaxation, as well as a deeper connection to yourself.

In this book, I have aimed to encapsulate all my knowledge, from the fundamentals of chair yoga, modifications and variations to support your practice, cultivating gratitude and mindfulness, a comprehensive 28-day challenge, and how to balance your physical and mental health. I hope that you feel motivated to apply all of these concepts as part of your new life.

As you continue your chair yoga practice, I encourage you to be patient and embrace each accomplishment, no matter how small it may look. Embark on this as a lifelong journey of self-discovery, where you discover something new about yourself that you never would have known if you didn't nurture your body and mind in this comprehensive way. May the wisdom and practices you've gained here serve as a source of inspiration, empowerment, and joy in your life. I wish you all the best in your ongoing pursuit of health, happiness, and a balanced, fulfilling life.

YOUR FEEDBACK MATTERS: LEAVE A REVIEW AND SHARE YOUR THOUGHTS

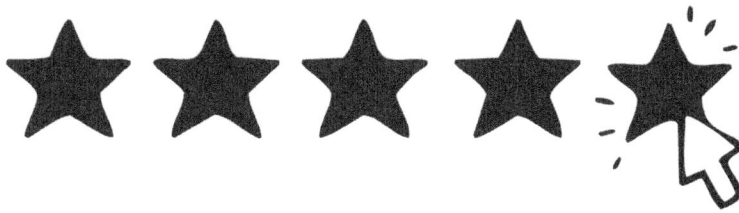

We are thrilled that you have chosen to read all the tips and information mentioned in this book as a companion to help you achieve a healthier and fitter body through chair yoga. We hope it brings value, enriches perspectives, and ignites the passion to achieve a more independent life thanks to a body that is comfortable to move around in. We greatly appreciate your support, and we hope you are enjoying your new book.

From Balanced Living Books, we plan to continue providing content that inspires as many people to live physically active and healthy lifestyles, and your opinion matters in this process. If you found this book enjoyable, inspiring, and helpful, kindly consider leaving a review and sharing your thoughts with others by scanning this QR code. Your feedback can make significant differences; both to help people out there discover the valuable benefits of this book and to allow us to continue offering content that resonates with what people need to stay healthy.

Scan the QR code or visit this URL to write a review on Amazon:
https://balancedlivingbooks.com/review-tb-cyfs60/

REFERENCES

Adra, S. (2019, August 12). Kapalbhati versus bhastrika: Comparing two powerful pranayama practices. Yogapedia. https://www.yogapedia.com/kapalbhati-versus-bhastrika-comparing-two-powerful-pranayama-practices/2/11580

Alkhatib, A. (2018, April 13). 6 yoga contraindications you need to know. Dumb Little Man. https://www.dumblittleman.com/yoga-contraindications/

Alternate nostril breathing: How & why to practice. (2022, September 7). Cleveland Clinic. https://health.clevelandclinic.org/alternate-nostril-breathing/

Amy. (2020, October 16). The meaning of savasana: Why we do this final yoga pose. Mind Body Badass. https://www.infiniteembers.com/what-is-savasana-meaning/

Anekwe, C., & Reddy, N. (2021, December 6). Yoga for weight loss: Benefits beyond burning calories. Harvard Health. https://www.health.harvard.edu/blog/yoga-for-weight-loss-benefits-beyond-burning-calories-202112062650

Ashish. (2020, June 12). Bhastrika pranayama (bellows breath): Benefits & how to do. Fitsri Yoga. https://www.fitsri.com/pranayama/bhastrika

Ashish. (2022, July 16). Surya mudra: Benefits, steps, precautions & side effects. Fitsri. https://www.fitsri.com/yoga-mudras/surya-mudra

Ayne, B. (2023). Chair yoga: Easy, healing yoga moves you can do with a chair. Emerson & Tilman Publishers.

Barnes, M. (2019, September 11). Is there a connection between junk food and mental health problems? Body+Mind Magazine. https://bodymind.com/junk-food-and-mental-health/

Bayly, K. (2022, November 20). 5 common yoga mistakes & how to fix them. T3. https://www.t3.com/features/yoga-mistakes-and-how-to-fix-them

Blair, M. (2011, November 23). 5 ways to express gratitude through yoga. Yoga Journal. https://www.yogajournal.com/practice/5-ways-express-gratitude-yoga/

Boggenpoel, E. (2021, October 7). 6 yoga myths debunked. Live Science. https://www.livescience.com/6-yoga-myths-debunked

Brennan, D. (2021, October 25). Mental benefits of walking. WebMD. https://www.webmd.com/fitness-exercise/mental-benefits-of-walking

Brill, J. (2018, October 11). 3 steps to modify prasarita padottanasana (wide-legged standing forward bend). Yoga Journal. https://www.yogajournal.com/poses/3-steps-to-modify-prasarita-padottanasana/

Burgin, T. (2020, September 1). How to choose the perfect yoga block . Yoga Basics. https://www.yogabasics.com/connect/yoga-blog/how-to-choose-the-perfect-yoga-block/

Burke, A. (n.d.). "If it hurts, don't do it": Considering pain and pain language in yoga. Yoga International. https://yogainternational.com/article/view/if-it-hurts-dont-do-it-considering-pain-and-pain-language-in-yoga/

Castle, T. (2020, October 27). 70 powerful quotes to motivate you to build good habits. Lifehack. https://www.lifehack.org/889488/habits-quotes

Chalicha, E. (2023, June 14). Does chair yoga work? The truth according to wellness experts. Better Me. https://betterme.world/articles/does-chair-yoga-work/

Cherry, K. (2020, May 13). What is consciousness? Verywell Mind. https://www.verywellmind.com/what-is-consciousness-2795922

Clay, R. (2017, September). The link between food and mental health. American Psychological Association. https://www.apa.org/monitor/2017/09/food-mental-health

Clear, J. (2018). Atomic habits : An easy and proven way to build good habits and break bad ones. Penguin Random House.

Common yoga myths and misconceptions . (2023, July 12). LifeMD. https://lifemd.com/learn/debunking-yoga-myths-and-misconceptions-separating-fact-from-fiction

Cunningham, S. (2018, September 19). Understanding breathing and the importance of taking a deep breath. UCHealth Today. https://www.uchealth.org/today/understanding-breathing-and-the-importance-of-taking-a-deep-breath/

Danao, K. (2022, August 10). 60 looking back quotes to see how far you've come. Quote Ambition. https://www.quoteambition.com/looking-back-quotes/

Derrick. (2021, May 25). Chair yoga for seniors - 17 great stretches. Elder Guru. https://www.elderguru.com/chair-yoga-for-seniors-17-great-stretches/

Do you need to be flexible to do yoga? (n.d.). Yoga Pose. Retrieved October 22, 2023, from https://yogapose.com/articles/do-you-need-to-be-flexible-to-do-yoga/

Drake, K. (2022, June 22). What is chair yoga? What are its benefits? GoodRx. https://www.goodrx.com/well-being/movement-exercise/chair-yoga

Erica. (2018, December 17). 18 different types of yoga props for beginners and advanced yogis. Yoga Baron. https://www.yoga-baron.com/yoga-props

Evans, C. (2005). Malnutrition in the elderly: a multifactorial failure to thrive. The Permanente Journal, 9(3), 38–41. https://doi.org/10.7812/tpp/05-056

Ezrin, S. (2021, November 18). Adaptive yoga: Making yoga accessible for every body. Healthline. https://www.healthline.com/health/fitness/adaptive-yoga

Fish pose. (n.d.). Ekhart Yoga. https://www.ekhartyoga.com/resources/yoga-poses/fish-pose

5 excuses to skip yoga (and reasons to stop making excuses). (2011, September 17). Yoga Journal. https://www.yogajournal.com/lifestyle/5-excuses-to-skip-yoga-class-and-reasons-to-stop-making-excuses/

Fletcher, J. (2020, November 25). How long can the average person hold their breath? Benefits and risks. Medical News Today. https://www.medicalnewstoday.com/articles/how-long-can-the-average-person-hold-their-breath

Fogoros, R. N. (2019). The role of the vagus nerve in the nervous system. Verywell Health. https://www.verywellhealth.com/vagus-nerve-anatomy-1746123

Frothingham , S. (2019, December 18). Ujjayi breathing for relaxation and relief. Healthline. https://www.healthline.com/health/fitness-exercise/ujjayi-breathing

Giubilaro, G. (2015, October 12). 3 ways to modify malasana + practice pratyahara. Yoga Journal. https://www.yogajournal.com/poses/modify-practice-pratyahara-malasana/

Goddess pose hands behind head side bend yoga (parsva utkata konasana hasta sirsa). (2020, March 5). Tummee. https://prelive-dot-tummee-prod.appspot.com/yoga-poses/goddess-pose-hands-behind-head-side-bend/

Goddess pose on chair arms down yoga (utkata konasana on chair hasta down) | Yoga sequences, benefits, variations, and Sanskrit pronunciation. (2020, February). Tummee. https://www.tummee.com/yoga-poses/goddess-pose-on-chair-arms-down

Golden Lion Publications. (2021). The new you: The only chair yoga for seniors guide you'll ever need.

Gotter, A. (2017, July 5). Visceral fat. Healthline. https://www.healthline.com/health/visceral-fat

Graham, B. (2022, June 23). Self-Care 101: Building better health habits - guides. The Paper Gown. https://www.zocdoc.com/blog/self-care-101-building-better-health-habits/

Guide to nutrition in older adults. (2021, February 21). Dispatch Health. https://www.dispatchhealth.com/blog/guide-to-nutrition-in-older-adults/

Hamrick, S. (2022). Chair yoga for seniors: Seated stretches and poses you can do anywhere to increase flexibility, mobility, balance, and strength.

Happy baby pose (ananda balasana). (2008, May 7). Yoga Journal. https://www.yogajournal.com/poses/happy-baby-pose/

Harvard Health Publishing. (2016, March 10). Learning diaphragmatic breathing. Harvard Health. https://www.health.harvard.edu/healthbeat/learning-diaphragmatic-breathing

Harvard School of Public Health. (2020, October 19). Calcium. The Nutrition Source; Harvard. https://www.hsph.harvard.edu/nutritionsource/calcium/

HealthyAtHome. (n.d.). WHO. https://www.who.int/campaigns/connecting-the-world-to-combat-coronavirus/healthyathome/healthyathome---healthy-diet

Helmer, J. (2022, February 16). Chair yoga poses: How to get started. WebMD. https://www.webmd.com/fitness-exercise/features/chair-yoga-poses

Herrington, S. (2021, October 20). Why is child's pose so insanely calming? Yoga Journal. https://www.yogajournal.com/poses/why-is-childs-pose-so-calming/

Hopes, S. (2023, August 28). Forget squats — this 20-minute chair yoga routine sculpts stronger legs and core muscles without weights. Tom's Guide. https://www.tomsguide.com/features/forget-squats-this-20-minute-chair-yoga-routine-sculpts-stronger-legs-and-core-muscles-without-weights

How to create a calm yoga space at home. (2020, December 4). Bliss Lights. https://blisslights.com/blogs/blisslights/how-to-create-a-calm-yoga-space-at-home

How to do kapalbhati pranayama | kapalbhati pranayama | skull shining breathing technique. (n.d.). Art of Living. https://www.artofliving.org/yoga/breathing-techniques/skull-shining-breath-kapal-bhati

How to get started with chair yoga. (n.d.). University of Arkansas. https://www.uaex.uada.edu/life-skills-wellness/health/physical-activity-resources/chair-yoga.aspx

Is it safe to hold your breath? (2023, April 29). WebMD. https://www.webmd.com/a-to-z-guides/is-it-safe-to-hold-your-breath#091e9c5e8216224e-1-2

James, R. (2021, February 26). The 10 best yoga breathing exercises. Awaken. https://awaken.com/2021/02/the-10-best-yoga-breathing-exercises/

Jeffries, T. Y. (2022, July 3). 13 chair yoga poses you can do without leaving your seat. Yoga Journal. https://www.yogajournal.com/yoga-101/types-of-yoga/chair-yoga-poses/

Kabe, K. (n.d.). Chair yoga for weight loss: How it works and why it's effective. The Power Yoga. https://thepoweryoga.com/chair-yoga-for-weight-loss-how-it-works/

Lakshmi Voelker, E-RYT500, C-IAYT, YACEP, owner of Lakshmi Voelker chair yoga, author. (n.d.). https://nancyslist.org/2019/03/29/lakshmi-voelker-e-ryt500-c-iayt-yacep-ayc-ambassador-and-chair-yoga/

Lehmkuhl, L. (2020). Chair yoga for seniors : Stretches and poses that you can do sitting down at home. Skyhorse Publishing.

List of all mudras. (2019, June 27). Yoga Mudra Step by Step and Its Benefits. https://coolmeditation.wordpress.com/list-of-all-mudras/

Lovett, S. (2022, May 16). Benefits of using essential oils with meditation. Base Formula. https://www.baseformula.com/blog/essential-oils-for-meditation

Lucchetti, L. (2023, September 12). Spine misalignment: What are some symptoms? Medical News Today. https://www.medicalnewstoday.com/articles/spine-misalignment-symptoms

Manaker, L. (2021, November 19). How does deep breathing improve your digestion? Verywell Health. https://www.verywellhealth.com/diaphragmatic-breathing-stress-digestion-5209648

McCaffrey, R., Taylor, D., Marker, C., & Park, J. (2019). A pilot study of the effects of chair yoga and chair-based exercise on biopsychosocial outcomes in older adults with lower extremity osteoarthritis. Holistic Nursing Practice, 33(6), 321–326. https://doi.org/10.1097/hnp.0000000000000355

McGinley, K. (2015, October 22). Why savasana is the hardest yoga pose. The Chopra Center. https://chopra.com/articles/why-savasana-is-the-hardest-yoga-pose

McGonigle, A. (2023, January 4). 4 ways to practice malasana. Yoga Journal. https://www.yogajournal.com/practice/ways-to-practice-malasana/

Mindful eating. (2020, September 14). The Nutrition Source; Harvard T.H. Chan, School of Public Health. https://www.hsph.harvard.edu/nutritionsource/mindful-eating/

Mironenko, C. (2021, July 30). Is yoga safe to do after joint replacement surgery? Hospital for Special Surgery. https://www.hss.edu/article_yoga-after-joint-replacement.asp

Nutrition. (2019). Harvard Health. https://www.health.harvard.edu/topics/nutrition

Olondriz, P. (2021, January 25). Background music for yoga classes. Legis Music. https://legismusic.com/background-music-yoga-classes

Panasevich, J. (2018, February 13). Why don't you do yoga? A comeback for every excuse. U.S. News. https://health.usnews.com/health-news/blogs/eat-run/articles/2018-02-13/why-dont-you-do-yoga-a-comeback-for-every-excuse

Pietrangelo, A. (2022, March 25). Anulom vilom pranayama: Potential benefits and how to practice it. Healthline. https://www.healthline.com/health/anulom-vilom-pranayama

Pizer, A. (2019). How asanas are used in yoga today. Verywell Fit. https://www.verywellfit.com/what-is-asana-3566793

Pizer, A. (2021, July 23). Easy pose must be done right for benefits. Verywell Fit. https://www.verywellfit.com/easy-pose-sukhasana-3567124

Q+A: Why do we set intentions in yoga? (2020, September 2). Yoga Journal. https://www.yogajournal.com/yoga-101/philosophy/qa-set-intentions-yoga

Quinn, S. (2022, February). The surprising benefits of eating together. BBC Food. https://www.bbc.co.uk/food/articles/eating_together

Raman, R. (2017, September 5). How your nutritional needs change as you age. Healthline. https://www.healthline.com/nutrition/nutritional-needs-and-aging

Ravishankar, R. A., & Alpaio, K. (2022, August 30). 5 ways to set more achievable goals. Harvard Business Review. https://hbr.org/2022/08/5-ways-to-set-more-achievable-goals

Reid, S. (2023, February 28). Gratitude: The benefits and how to practice it . Help Guide. https://www.helpguide.org/articles/mental-health/gratitude.htm

Revolved goddess pose yoga (parivrtta utkata konasana). (n.d.). Tummee. https://www.tummee.com/yoga-poses/revolved-goddess-pose